Something to Think About

Some Unbelievably Basic
Ideas About Nutrition

NutritionLuke

authorHOUSE®

AuthorHouse™
1663 Liberty Drive
Bloomington, IN 47403
www.authorhouse.com
Phone: 1 (800) 839-8640

Published by AuthorHouse 07/27/2015

ISBN: 978-1-5049-2461-0 (sc)
ISBN: 978-1-5049-2460-3 (e)

Library of Congress Control Number: 2015911791

Print information available on the last page.

Contents

Ideas are the most powerful thing a person can influence. To anyone from Hitler to Einstein, ideas have the potential to spark a change in civilization. The "idea" of the internet literally revolutionized the human species. Facebook is a great example of an idea that changed how people communicate. The idea of gravity turned out to be What governs all modern physics.

Ideas are provoked by something: an influence of some sort. Quantum mechanics attempts to explain that a thought occurs which then causes a physical reaction of a neurotransmitter to release chemicals to then stimulate the brain and tell it what to do with that thought or realization. This is awesome; however, it still doesn't explain the root cause of where the thought originated.

What inspires ideas? Where did I get the influence to write this book? Why am I driven to spread knowledge and provoke thought? I simply think that there is no greater reason for us to be on this planet than to help each other. If I have an idea or an out-of-the-box thought that could potentially help others, wouldn't it be against my purpose here on this planet to not express this idea?

I don't know. I really don't, and nobody does. One thing I can say is that ideas are more powerful than the most powerful weapon of destruction or any cure for cancer. Ideas are behind all of the great and horrible things in this life.

I hope with this book that I inspire thought. There are enough "experts" out there to read. We all have an app on our phone of our favorite search engine to use to look up info. This is not the problem. The problem is that as a society we rely on what we are told and simply don't question anything.

For example: a doctor recommends a prescription for your mental health. Do you ask what this medication does? Not what the label says it can be prescribed for, but how does it work, what does it do to the brain? Is there anything else natural that does the same thing? If you do not get an answer or someone who is supposed to be an "expert" does not explain why or how, then should you really be taking that medication?

In my individual sessions with clients I try my best to explain why I make a recommendation. There are many different theories and interpretations of research to choose from when making a recommendation. One book says look at the pH content of food, the other says eat high fat, then low fat, then gluten free - either way, a change is being implemented from your current diet because your current lifestyle is negatively affecting your life. Why do I look so much into the relationship between clients and food? All they want is a "diet," and I'm over here asking about childhood traditions. However, when the client and I establish that sugary treats were the reward for doing something good, the client cannot ignore the correlation between overeating sweets as an adult and the "good" feeling associated with the childhood treat.

Again, just something to provoke thought: something to think about.

The following is a collection of blog posts developed over a year of continued education, personal transformation, and application with my clients. My purpose in presenting a variety of ideas and perspectives here is to allow me to touch base with a wide range of people and educate those who otherwise would not have access to this information.

I was raised in a small town in Nebraska where education regarding nutrition was lacking to say the least. Even when I got to college and began my first nutrition studies, I realized that nutrition was a topic that continues to evolve, and new research is always coming out. I also realized that with all of the different topics (and majors) I attempted in college, nutrition and helping people always continued to be a passion in my life.

Through this book, I want to help people continue to learn and grow in their own lives. My nutritional practices incorporate a strong mental health emphasis because there is more to health than just, "eat this not that."

I believe food is a medicine that can help people in so many ways. The more you know and the more you are willing to challenge rigid behaviors, the more useful nutrition information can be. For example, chicken is a good source of lean protein; however, if I tell you that fish is also a good protein source with other "outside" benefits, then you can improve on your decision and overall health with this additional information. Again, immediate change is minimal, but consistency over time allows the body to change noticeably. Maybe you can even lose stubborn body fat, reduce inflammation, and, to be quite honest, prevent the occurrence of diseases.

The body is a very unique and amazing organism, yet people have decided to reconstruct the workings of the body by engineering and chemically altering the foods we eat. People tend to want to categorize and control something that it is ever-changing, rather than stepping back, looking at the big picture, and moving on.

Ah, now I do have an advantage in that I am a psychotherapist with a strong nutritional background as opposed to solely being a nutritionist. In fact, research shows that nutritional education alone doesn't change behaviors. For example, I know that pizza tastes good and no matter how much information I get on the detriments of eating it, it still stimulates my brain in a way that very few things can.

With my own clients, I want them to implement a behavior modification where the client views their relationship with food as a rational experience where nutrients exist instead of just pleasure, where we appreciate and love ourselves enough to want the best that health and wellness have to offer us.

Confidence and self-respect is evident in people who take pride in what they do. If a man is working on his craft, he is comfortable in his realm. If a businesswoman is negotiating a business deal, then she may feel most assured there. I personally feel most comfortable when I eat healthy, think healthy, and do whatever I can to help others.

This book is a combination of several passions of mine. I love to write (nobody promised you the second coming of Malcolm Gladwell here), help people, research, learn, and find ways to interpret and apply information. So, please enjoy the most recent year and a half of ideas and concepts of health, both- mental and physical-with a touch of humor, and no matter what your current perspective, consider these ideas for what they are …"Something to Think About …"

Cheat Day May Be Killing You!

As sad as it is to say, I am going to have to start this post off by announcing a loss to the family:

cheat day.

We all know what I am talking about: the day of the week when we overindulge in foods we would not normally allow ourselves to eat—for physical appearances, of course.

Just in case there are some people who do not implement a cheat day, it goes something like this:

Monday: chicken and broccoli
Tuesday: tuna and sweet potato
Wednesday: egg-white omelet and oatmeal
Thursday: chicken and broccoli (again)
Friday: protein shake and raw almonds
Saturday: pizza, wings, ice cream, chips, cheese nachos, doughnuts, cookies, licorice, sub sandwiches, etc. Veggies? Don't you dare on a cheat day!
Sunday: oatmeal and boiled eggs

I am telling you that people will deprive themselves all week so that they can cheat on their diets on a chosen weekend day. Why do we need to have a cheat day?

When it comes to foods, especially enticing ones that we cannot wait to eat on special occasions, a cheat day may not be beneficial for your goals. Consider this possibility: a food addiction is really no different from a drug addiction except that the substances are legal and socially encouraged. Seriously, you would never help a crack addict stay clean for six days a week and then encourage him or her to cheat on his or her sobriety on a Friday night.

It makes no sense that we reward ourselves with food because we ate what we were supposed to be eating all week anyway. Nobody rewards the guy who made the clothes we wear because they fit us. I rarely get a pat on the back for just showing up.

No. It's what is just expected.

Eating unprocessed foods without a cheat day is essential for optimal health. One day of processed foods can ruin your digestive tract and the many benefits gained from eating healthy for weeks — maybe even years, according to some researchers. Some studies found in popular books, such as *Wheat Belly* and *Grain Brain*, claim the detriments can last up to ten years!

When a person consumes highly processed foods made of sugar, flour, trans fat, and other rancid and processed ingredients, it stresses the body. This makes for a difficult recovery, whether you physically feel it or not.

Well, scarf down that pizza and enjoy that sub sandwich. Shoot, throw in some chips made with hydrogenated oil, because it may take until your last days on earth to fully process out the negative effects of your "reward."

I also like to reward myself for doing a good job in school by dropping a bowling ball on my foot and then giving my body the full amount of time to heal.

Remind yourself that the human body does not need processed sugars or fats, no matter how badly you convince yourself that it does as you spend forty-five minutes picking out the perfect cheat foods in the grocery store. (I know people who do that.) This is a mental craving that I compare to what drug addicts go through every day, as in you do not need this highly processed drug of a frozen pizza. Instead, stick to your diet rich in vitamins, minerals, enzymes, and all of the various benefits found in whole-food items. The rewards of increased energy and improved health will be more than enough.

Also, I recommend looking up new and innovative ways to eat the same healthy foods you like. The Internet is full of recipes.

Granola: It's a Dessert!

Have you ever looked at a granola package? Whether or not you are interested in going on a long hike, mountain biking, or doing a triathlon, granola is there for you. In most cases, examples of high-level activities are what I see on granola packages and commercials.

Shoot, why not eat granola? I mean granola tastes amazing, and all of the dried fruits and nuts are so much sweeter than when you eat them by themselves. Plus, if we categorize foods into good and bad categories, granola is definitely in the "good" category.

I mean it's 100 percent natural, according to the marketing departments!

Here's the deal: granola (God bless it) has been glorified way too long. I want this post to inform people about the dark side of granola to prevent this snack from being one of your choices of foods to eat.

Facts: Granola has 453 calories per cup, including twelve grams of fat (not bad) and twenty-eight grams of good ol' sugar, with a total of eighty grams of carbohydrates per serving. The nutrition label says it all.

Just absorb these numbers for a minute, and then ask yourself if that is what you thought they were. Most of society puts this positive spin on granola as if it were some kind of miracle energy drug. The truth is it is a lot of readily available energy. So much in fact that your body then has plenty to store in the adipose tissues of the body.

Fact: One McDonald's Big Mac sandwich has 590 calories, thirty-four grams of fat (eleven of which are saturated), and eight grams of sugar out of the total forty-seven carbs. To be fair to the Big Mac, on paper, it does contain twenty-four grams of protein per sandwich, but the "meat" quality is so low that who knows if you are actually getting twenty-four grams of *usable* protein?

Interestingly, people's assumptions about these two food items are that they exist on opposite ends of the healthy food spectrum.

Granola is supposed to be the healthy example and part of a nutritious diet and the Big Mac is on the opposite end, setting the example for pure crap.

Then why are these two food items so closely related in terms of calories, with granola having almost double the total amount of carbs, three times the amount of sugar, and none of the protein?

Granola is not a good choice when it comes to choosing a healthy snack — pure and simple.

Healthy snacks still need to be foods that are as unprocessed as possible. I understand that many different types of granola can be manufactured many different ways with varying amounts of sugars, but it is still highly processed sugar. My question here is this: when was the last time you read about ancient Roman societies eating cranberry granola or — better yet — growing granola trees?

It doesn't matter how something is packaged and sold or the health claims on the brightly colored package. If it is not naturally grown, and the product contains unwanted grains and sugars, it can lead to excess fat very quickly through activating a rapid and overwhelming insulin response.

Word of advice: if something is packaged as "nutritious" but has to be explained why it is good for you, then most likely it is not.

High-fructose corn syrup, with which more and more people are becoming familiar, was even advertised as being "not that bad for you" in some commercials that compared it to sugar. Do not get it wrong: high-fructose corn syrup is bad for you and contains zero nutrients that the body needs for survival. These sugars are so devoid of nutrients that they actually leave the body at a deficit as they pull nutrients from the body during digestion, not to mention the strain put on the liver to digest. Ever heard of non-alcoholic fatty-liver disease?

Interestingly, this "sugar" also is the ingredient that is found in so many packages and different brands of granola that people love to eat as a "healthy" snack.

To sum it up, unless you are about to run a triathlon or go on a fifty-mile bike ride, say no to the snack with simple sugars containing more than half a day's worth of carbohydrate intake in a cup.

Sugar, Sugar Everywhere

Sugar has many names: barley malt, beet sugar, brown sugar, buttered syrup, cane-juice crystals, cane sugar, caramel, corn syrup, corn-syrup solids, confectioner's sugar, carob syrup, castor sugar, date sugar, dextrin, dextrose, fructose, fruit juice, fruit-juice concentrate, galactose, glucose, glucose solids, golden sugar, golden syrup, grape sugar, high-fructose corn syrup, honey, icing sugar, invert sugar, lactose, maltodextrin, maltose, malt syrup, maple syrup, molasses, raw sugar, refiner's syrup, rice syrup, sorbitol, sucrose, turbinado sugar, yellow sugar, etc.

Well *boooowdy!* That is a lot of ways to interpret crap! Don't get me wrong: some of these named sugars are less processed than others are, some have lower glycemic ratings, and some are sort of found in nature. Regardless, the way we are consuming them in our society is just scary.

So we can clearly see that there is enough sugar, or at least sugar by-products, available to keep Americans obese for years to come. Shoot, it might even worsen the "epidemic," as it has been labeled now. Every year, we hear stats about heart disease and how it kills more people than anything else does; however, let us take a step back and ask ourselves, "What is causing heart disease?"

Saturated fats! Beef products! Hormones! Stress! Smoking!

While these are contributing factors, more and more research is being released and reanalyzed to show that sugar, in its multiple forms, may be the single-most leading cause of heart disease.

Here is why. When we consume sugar, our body releases insulin to help break down this readily available form of energy into glucose, and in many instances (and depending on how processed the foods are that we are eating), more and more insulin has to be released to help lower the body's blood sugar levels.

Simply put, if you eat a high-carbohydrate meal, insulin is released to remove glucose from the blood. The leftover glucose then converts to glycogen that is stored in the liver and muscles for energy use, resulting in an enzyme (with a name too long to mention) that is released to convert blood sugar to fat!

When carbohydrates are consumed and digested, glycerol phosphate is introduced into the system, free-flowing fatty acids are scooped up, and triglycerides are formed and stored in adipose tissue. See? Without the carbohydrates, your body can't make triglycerides to store in the adipose tissue.

During the primitive days of mankind we needed every available resource to keep blood sugars up. The high blood sugar levels and weight gain were stored in the body as excess energy that was regularly used thus preventing vessel-damaging blood sugar floating in the body's blood stream. The same process does not work well with today's more sedentary lifestyles.

So simply summarizing here: SUGAR IN ALL ITS DIFFERENT VARIETIES IS NOTHING MORE THAN A SUBSTANCE THAT TRIGGERS THE BRAIN TO CONTINUE EATING ALL THE WHILE LEECHING NUTRIENTS NEEDED FOR DIGESTION OF ESSENTIAL COMPOUNDS!!!

See, the correct choice of all the sugars would be: none!

Alcoholic or Carboholic?

Some recent research has led me to the idea that alcoholics may not necessarily be addicted to the intoxicating effects of alcohol as much as they are addicted to the effects of the sugar content in alcohol.

Remember, carbohydrates are taken in for energy. Well, because sugars burn very fast you need to continue feeding with sugar if that is your preferred form of energy (aka America diets). Now let's think about what alcohol really is: the most available and fastest reacting sugar out there. So when alcoholics begin drinking they are feeding their bodies these sugars, usually in high amounts too. The body then begins signaling a "craving" during periods of sobriety or any period of time that it has gone too long without sugar.

The next day after an alcohol binge the physiological withdrawal effects (resulting mostly from the intoxicating effects) become apparent. The body craves more sugar due to the hypoglycemic after-effects created as a result of a devastating night of sugars and dancing.

Put gas on a fire and it doesn't burn that bright for very long before it needs more fuel: this is exactly how the body and alcohol work. Not only does the body want more, but it needs to recharge due to ethanol's damaging effects and the resulting low blood sugar.

Alcoholics tend to experience "cravings," which are different than the desire or want to escape reality. This is a physiological effect of the body wanting sugars that it has not received during an extended period of sobriety. To make matters worse, many addicts also have poor diets that put the body into a cycle of craving. Unfortunately, in a moment of weakness the signal of wanting sugar gets misplaced as a "craving" for alcohol. This could occur due to the sugar found in sweets, like added sugar in coffee that is no longer satisfying. The body is then left in a state of distress aka craving.

After a night of drinking, ask yourself why you crave fast, processed foods the next day instead of, say, a vegetable and protein stir fry? Even some of the most dedicated healthy eaters crumble during a hangover. Why? Because the body craves those sugars again, and this time the sugars from a processed meal will have to do.

A way to prevent a "craving" is to first, foremost, and forever, sober up.

Secondly- instead of feeding the body sugars that it then converts to glucose- let us feed it fats for energy. This prevents the release of insulin and stops unused glucose from running amuck in the blood stream. High fat diets containing moderate protein offer the best and most efficient way to fulfill the body's energy needs.

Research, which is still being conducted, has shown that by changing the diets of recovering alcoholics cravings are significantly reduced leading to more satisfying lives. In this case, all health aspects are factored into recovery, not just sobriety.

Every day I work with and watch clients drink soda, eat candy, smoke cigarettes, and fulfill every other addiction besides the one for which they are in treatment. These cross addictive tendencies are nothing more than maladaptive coping skills that continue to keep the client's mind on the brink of a relapse.

Just because a person is no longer using a substance does not mean that they are any healthier!

Breakfast, You're My Only Friend!

I get asked by multiple people a week (randomly, mind you) to assist them with their health and nutrition goals (usually weight loss). One of the first things I ask (besides telling them to cut out fast foods, soda, and beer) is "do you eat breakfast"?

The importance of breakfast in determining how the rest of your day will go cannot be stressed enough. When you consume breakfast, you not only kick start your metabolism but kick start your digestive process as well.

This next part I believe is more important: when people skip meals throughout the day, especially breakfast, the internal digestive organs get a little "off." Being "off" can result in a number of difficulties, especially for the millions of people in the U.S. who deal with digestive problems. Being "off" means that your body is set to start the digestive process later in the day, moving everything else later, hence late night food cravings. It is like you have reset your clock a few hours back so even though it is night time, your internal clock still thinks it is eating time.

Many people think that the first thing to do to lose weight is to stop eating.

"Well, if I am not taking in calories then my body will burn off this fat,"- Young Luke (he wasn't the brightest).

This could not be further from the truth. I may have already said this before, but it is worth repeating again: eating breakfast is literally the first step of the day to a healthier and more in-control you. After breakfast we can talk about sensible lunches, snacks, late night snacks etc., but first we have to wake up and eat breakfast.

"But I am not hungry in the morning," my fiancé and pretty much anyone who skips breakfast says.

This occurs because you have trained your body to eat later in the day; therefore you're eating into the late hours of the evening. What sense does it make for your brain to send hunger signals if it is not going to get anything? Don't worry though: your body will always send signals of hunger later on in the day and into the late night to make up for those lost calories. Unless you train your body to expect something in the morning, preferably protein and a complex carbohydrate source such as oatmeal or Greek yogurt, it will never get used to regular eating times and that "hunger" in the evening will continue to linger. My fiancé has figured out the pleasure of protein shakes and finds them convenient when she does not have very much time or feels little hunger in the morning.

As for the night time? Go to bed and get needed rest. Then, as with any other engine, jumpstart it in the morning with BREAKFAST!!!

I Can't Fight This ...
(mmmmm pumpkin) ... Feeling Anymore

I'm not sure if it's the cooler weather, the leaves changing, or the fact that I was able to wear a jacket to work for the first time this week that led me to crave those seasonal foods rich in useless and processed carbohydrates. Maybe it was the overwhelming aisles of Halloween candy at the stores or maybe it's because I was raised in a household that glorified the changing of the seasons with food.

Whew, that felt good to get off my chest.

The truth is, I pride myself on recognizing my own body and why it craves certain types of foods. As I realized, lately it has been such a constant craving for breads, cookies, and cakes (you know, the good stuff) that I have to question why.

Now, this post really goes out to people who are trying to lose weight or, like me, just like to live a healthy lifestyle. From my recent posts, eating breads, starches, cookies, and all the "good" stuff doesn't correlate with a healthy lifestyle, plain and simple. So why now would I be writing to say that I am craving such things?

Because it happens.

In many instances when your body begins to crave a food, it is because there is a nutrient missing in your diet. For example, when people go on crash diets they most often begin to crave everything under the sun. Another example is when people eat no carbs: all they want is breads, but if they incorporated some veggies, legumes, or whole grains they would feel more satisfied.

Eat breakfast: check

Workout: check

Eat veggies: check

Eat healthier fats: check

I even started adding the supplement Glutamine by putting a scoop of powder underneath my tongue during sweet cravings. One of Glutamine's functions is that it can alter sweet cravings. It absorbs faster when put under your tongue. However, I did not really feel any relief from the craving, even after thirty minutes.

I already eat seven to eight meals a day, so you know I am not starving myself.

As I touched on earlier, growing up I lived with the "Queen of the Baked Goods" Kathie Meier (aka mom). This lady can bake cookies, breads, cookie bars, cheesecakes, and – worse yet – she enjoys doing it. Needless to say as an adolescent I had access to all the finest pastries and desserts. Hence my two hundred and fifteen pound frame in 6th grade.

The point here is that even though you can eat the best foods, workout, and consume significant amounts of whole nutrients, there are still going to be those days where, for whatever reason, you just want a cookie, or in my case, five.

Remind yourself that when you are intensely craving processed foods, it is not your body's way of letting you know you NEED them, but an emotional response to "crave" the pleasure which can be fulfilled by sweets.

A lesson for many of us who struggle with sweet- tasting foods is that consuming a sweet is no way to fight a craving.

Giving in to desires will establish a pattern of a pleasure response to distress and intensify future cravings.

Pumpkins! (So Cliché)

Well, it's been that time of year now for about two weeks. In case you didn't notice the lattés at Starbucks, seasonal beers at the restaurants, or flavors being presented on Pinterest, it is definitely pumpkin season.

Pumpkins are good for you. They look pretty, we can cook their seeds, we can make pies, and we can even carve out and use every bit of the pulp.

Some health benefits of pumpkin include:

- Rich in antioxidants including alpha-carotene and beta-carotene, which give this fall vegetable its orange color.
- High in fiber. One cup of pumpkin meat contains three grams of dietary fiber.
- Low in calories (and fat). Minus all of the added sugar and butter, one cup of pumpkin contains only forty-nine calories.
- A good source of vitamin A, pumpkin also contains high amounts of vitamins C and E, magnesium, potassium, and iron.

Pumpkin also tastes good in pies, lattés, or even mellow crème form, such as in the bags of candy (my favorite form of pumpkin).

As much as people like the actual flavor of pumpkin, it seems we are resistant to eating it in its purest form, choosing instead to add butter, sugar, and other ingredients to make it more palatable.

Think about it: nobody eats pure pumpkin. Never have I sat down to a meal that includes pulp scooped out of a pumpkin. I have seen where you can buy pumpkin spice at any grocery store and add it to foods, however actual pumpkin is rarely used.

Growing up, the only time I saw pumpkin being used was when my mom would add cans of pumpkin to her breads, pies, or cheesecakes. Even when my mom made food from "scratch," I never saw her use the pulp from an actual pumpkin. Maybe it's the shell you are supposed to use. I don't really know.

I do know that what comes out of a can is said to be real pumpkin, and, depending on how it's processed, it is supposed to have the benefits listed above.

However, as with anything processed, a lot of antioxidants and vitamins can be burned off and may only benefit the truly raw pumpkin eaters among us. Sorry folks: big business sold us on nutrition again. More than likely the pumpkin we are all used to is processed desserts, or some Sara Lee knock off.

Trip to the Doctor

Recently, I had the good fortune to get an annual checkup from a very wise physician. While the thought of a doctor's office can sometimes induce nightmares about shots, stitches, being cut open and sick people, it is also a place where I get a lot of my references.

This office was quiet, clean and comfortable. There were even (dare I say it) pamphlets in the office on the importance of proper nutrition.

No way! What in the world would eating healthy have to do with a doctor's office visit?

Well, enough with the sarcasm. The answer is everything.

Nutrition is kind of my thing and I respect anybody who takes a stance on the value of eating proper nutrients in moderate amounts. Even if evidence may disprove what people think about vegan diets, juice diets, or just diets in general, those people, admirably, still took a stance.

Here was this doctor's stance: eat fruits and veggies with a healthy protein source for every meal and incorporate healthy fats in the evening instead of carbohydrates.

AAAAHHHHH!!!!

What? Where's the recommended magic pharmaceutical pill, surgery, or all liquid diet? Why can't the doctor write me a prescription, I follow it, and poof! Easy, healthy life?

By eating healthier, in moderate portions, a person can prolong his life with minimal cost: this seems to be the general consensus. So why wouldn't a doctor recommend healthy eating, even though he has little to gain if people were to actually make this change?

I respect the fact that the pamphlet didn't sugar coat eating properly, but explained what breads and processed carbohydrates can do to a body. The program I was reading about did not recommend a specific, doctor formulated protein source or any "us-only" supplement; instead, it highly recommended moderate amounts of egg whites and animal meats.

The idea of incorporating vegetables in some people's diets can honestly be too much to handle, so they turn away. This pamphlet explained the benefits of vitamins and antioxidants found in various veggies and how readily available they are in this form.

More and more doctors are getting on board with this whole nutrition thing. The days of prescribing a pill to solve all of your woes have to be realized for what it is: a phony hope. Under this thought process, if a pill could just burn up forty-five pounds of straight fat, what is stopping it from just eating through your whole body?

Putting gas in a car makes it run, but without it - or with the wrong kind (Ethanol 85, diesel, um... jet fuel) - the car simply won't run. If the body does not get its proper fuel (vitamins, minerals, proteins, fats, water) then it will not run efficiently either, or at all. The body is a little more advanced than a car engine and will do its best to accomplish all functions needed to sustain life as long as it can. However, if you are putting crap in your body (processed foods, sugar, trans-fat, excess vegetable oils, etc.), then you are now making the jobs of the GI tract, heart, lungs, lymph nodes, brain, skin, etc., very difficult. In the long run your engine will burn out quicker, as opposed to operating as a well energized machine meant to last.

As the pamphlet said, and yes there were some sales involved, eating properly is the only way to live a healthy life. Without the raw material your body needs to keep rebuilding itself and sustain this precious life we have, you can expect more medical bills, pills, and a lower quality of life due to various disorders and diseases caused by poor nutrition.

Very cool!

Happy Halloween Obesity!

I have a scary story for you about a disease that kills more people than any other disease. On top of that, there is a plague that can cause permanent blindness and your feet to swell to three times their normal size before you finally lose the limbs and ultimately die. There is also a virus that causes people to blow up like balloons and, because they grow so large, they often cannot be transported to the hospital for treatment and die.

AAAAHHHHHH, what could this possibly be?

Heart disease, diabetes, and obesity aka Metabolic Syndrome! Scary, huh?

For most people, Halloween brings memories of candy, parties, costumes, and haunted houses.

Of course I am going to ignore all of the other aspects of Halloween and focus directly on the candy.

I am not exactly sure when candy became so prevalent in American society, and honestly I don't feel like cheating to look it up right now. However, my guess is that candy started to become popular when high fructose corn syrup (HFCS) was invented back in 1977. Yes, high fructose corn syrup was invented. This is true because it was discovered in a laboratory and now allows for sweet foods to be made cheaply. Let us add a fat to the mix that mimics saturated fat and never gets old (trans fats) and we now have what we call today's "candy."

It does not matter if your favorite candy is Reese's, Snickers, Milky Way, Dots, Starbursts, or anything else found in the Halloween aisle at your local retailer. It is all made with pretty much the same ingredient: HFCS as far as the eye can see!

When a child goes trick-or-treating and comes home with pounds of candy to snack on for the next month, this can create a big problem.

Low quality ingredients create access to massive amounts of candy and may lead children to lose appreciation for these once-a-year treats.

When I was a child and left the houses where dental floss was the "treat," I would mutter some inappropriate words under my breath. It was like the biggest kick in the pants to not get a handful of candy. Then when I got home I would throw out all the candy I didn't like. Obviously Reese's made the cut; it was the little orange and black ones I never liked - the Mary Janes.

The point here is that because we have allowed society to overindulge for so long, we have encouraged the food industry to use the cheapest food ingredients and inventions to meet the ever-growing demand while making large profits. Unfortunately, the demand for sweet products will never be fully met and new addicts are being born every day. In the process, we created metabolic syndrome that consists of obesity, heart disease, and diabetes to name a few of the scary monsters.

Parents, do your kids a favor this Halloween and try to limit their candy intake after the holiday. Remember that just because it was given to them doesn't mean they have to have it all. When you limit their intake of candy, it makes for a higher appreciation of the candy they do get.

Why Sugar Makes You Sad

Let's start this one with a couple of facts:

1. The pleasure you experience when you do anything is controlled by the release and uptake of the neurotransmitters serotonin, dopamine and norepinephrine.
2. These neurotransmitters are made from amino acids.
3. Abundant amounts of amino acids are found in high-quality, protein-based products such as fish, beef, chicken, and eggs.
4. Processed carbohydrates, rancid oils, and fats used in food processing actually interfere with the ability of amino acids to be converted to neurotransmitters.

So essentially by eating a low-quality, highly- processed carbohydrate diet you may actually decrease the release of neurotransmitters signaling pleasure thereby lowering your quality of life.

It is interesting to note how depression and anxiety cases are on par with the rise of obesity and heart disease, signifying underlying causes to both mental and physical health problems.

Consuming massive amounts of various types of sugars and sweeteners not only interferes with our weight and appearance, but how we feel on the inside. People need to grasp the idea that by changing their diets to include more vegetables, moderate amounts of quality protein sources (preferably from meat), and healthy fat sources (fish, nuts, coconut oils, olive oils, grass fed butter), they can better improve the overall quality of their lives by way of mental health, weight loss, and higher energy levels just to name a few.

Break Yo Self ... ... Fool!

Truthfully, I just wanted to use that line from <u>Don't be a Menace</u>, but hopefully opinions about me and my intelligence aren't based on my preference for that movie alone.

That line reminds me of what most people do to their bodies every single day. WE break ourselves with the constant stress and anxiety we put our bodies through. Post after post here I am talking about what we should be eating and that our bodies were never meant to process the foods we do feed it. The body was also never meant to handle the constant stress we put it through.

Think about the last time you did not have a worry or care in the world.

Either people are striving to succeed in this ever-competitive world, or people are deciding to give up and accept their position in life where they never fully meet their goals. I respect the people who accept being content and enjoy life, but still there are constant stressors such as work, children, bills, chores, food, etc. No matter what your life consists of, stressors are what can keep you going or tear you down.

Eating a healthy diet is important to your overall mental health.

In my last post, I mentioned some facts about how healthy eating can lead to higher amounts of the neurotransmitters serotonin, norepinephrine, and dopamine. These again are released and reabsorbed by neurons in the brain when contentment and pleasure are aroused. Truth is, when people get stressed out, sleepy, hungry, or just plain stop taking care of themselves, the neurotransmitters are no longer being utilized as they should. In turn we are essentially breaking ourselves by our own poor choices.

Stress is all around us. Every day there is some challenge placed in front of us or some inner thoughts and processes that we need to deal with. If issues are consuming your life, please see a mental health practitioner for assistance. For some home remedies to better increase your quality of life, consume more fish, almonds (raw if you can), and green veggies for a good start. Even if a person chooses to eat poorly, then he will at least give the body the materials it needs to build neurotransmitters in the first place and keep the body content.

Dropping Acid Like the '60s

First things first: gluten is an incomplete protein usually found in the wheat sources that make up carbohydrates. Gluten also has been derived from and used in everything from hand soaps to lip balms.

When a person consumes gluten, it increases the sulfuric acid in the linings of the stomach and esophagus.

When acid content rises, the body is forced to balance it with a more alkaline product, such as calcium from the bones. Processed diets are usually low in fruits, vegetables, beans, or nuts (which are alkaline), all of which are needed to counterbalance the acidic food we consume (meat, sodas, and, of course, wheat being the worst) and maintain a balanced pH level in the body naturally.

The standard pH of a body is set at 7.4 and if it increases or decreases by as little as .5, it results in death.

Bones in the human body will literally turn to mush before allowing the pH level to increase much from the set 7.4. The image is much like when Frosty the Snowman melts because it is too hot (I needed a Christmas reference). The more gluten, sodas and other acidic products people consume and the fewer vegetables they eat to counteract the pH levels in the body, the harder the body works (including depleting the calcium stores, the bones) to balance.

A way to prevent the bones from becoming weak and brittle is to eat a balanced diet consisting of meats, vegetables, and healthy fats. Do not consume calcium supplements (because they hardly do anything anyway, low absorption and all) but commit to eating fewer processed and wheat-containing foods.

All along (and this will be a recurring theme throughout these blog posts) the government and its agencies have tried to use a food pyramid or some other recommendation to sell people on how carbs, including whole grains, need to make up the bulk of their calories. However, "whole" grains also are being misinterpreted as refined flours fortified with nutrients. More and more, refined flours are the very substances that are being held responsible for causing diabetes as well as increasing acidity in the body to such a degree that instances of osteoporosis and arthritis are increasing.

I Am Thankful for …
Overindulgence, I Guess!

The most annoying part of Thanksgiving - or Christmas for that matter - is that I continue to get a lot of questions about what a person can do for a diet or workout plan, but then they follow it with, "well, I'll start in January."

I do not know about you, but I hate clichés and beginning a diet or workout plan in January is so cliché.

Let us be honest, yes Thanksgiving is this week, I am very excited to go home and spend time with my family, but it does not mean that everything I have worked for physically has to turn to garbage because the holiday commercials and brightly colored lights are up.

My fiancé and friends will tell you that I am HUGE into the holiday season and wish I could take the month off work to enjoy all of it, but sadly I cannot. I must continue to show up to work, pay bills, maybe even work a little more so I can buy better presents for loved ones. All of this is great but somehow it appears that people cannot control themselves with desserts and treats and therefore overindulge.

Yes, there are a lot more temptations and yes, there are a lot more social events where people feel inclined and even encouraged to overindulge. Usually social gatherings consist of some simple carbohydrates dipped into an artificial cheese sauce or sugar. One cannot deny a sugar shaped Santa, but then, people feel bad about themselves and complain about lower energy levels leading to a higher likelihood of depression (a theory of mine due to hearing about it repeatedly).

I think as a society we have allowed ourselves to be at the mercy of overindulgence so much that it is now the reason for the season for many people. Cookies, cakes, candies, and crème brûlée (and that's only the good-tasting C words) are everywhere. Just like our pocketbooks, society is telling us to go into debt with our health because it is a certain time of year.

Once January hits, despite what the Mayan Calendar might say, we all torture ourselves with high expectations for weight loss and diets that usually end up being harder on our body than all of the overly-processed sugars and fats we consumed.

Enjoy the holiday season, along with other pleasurable activities and friends and family. If alone, enjoy just being alive and look forward to all of the possibilities for the upcoming year. Please do not put an extra 5-10 pounds of fat on just because of the constant temptations during the holiday season. Reserve your overindulgence when it is really warranted on the specific day: Thanksgiving and Christmas. Other than that, keep a tighter watch on your pocketbooks and maintain regular healthy diets: you will have less to pay back in early spring.

Put That Cookie Down!

One of my favorite Christmas movies is *Jingle all the Way* starring the one and only Arnold Schwarzenegger. One of my favorite lines in the movie is when Arnold yells through the phone at his nosy neighbor played by Phil Hartman to "put that cookie down!"

When I was a child, I thought because it was Christmas time, overindulgence was unavoidable. It was just something that a person did. Mom would bake Christmas cookies the entire month of December, and, of course, I was there to taste-test every single one, not to mention steal them for a snack.

I remember all of the school holiday parties and work functions as I got older. I remember hearing the statistics about the amount of weight people put on during the holidays until it seemed like it just happened - there was no way to control or prevent it. I figured that the people who kept the holiday weight off were the less fortunate who did not have any money for Christmas overindulgence.

Now I understand that, for the most part, nothing "just happens" to your body without some sort of influence. Even something as severe as cancer can be attributed to actions leading up to that point allowing for the cancerous cells to grow. Unfortunately for your waistline through the holiday season there are many, many more indulgences on a daily basis that really need to be ignored.

Imagine that made from scratch Christmas cookie full of Christmas cheer and happiness. Well, unfortunately it also is full of gluten, sugar, and in many cases trans-fat. Yes, I know, I sound like the Grinch when I break down the happiness and innocence of Christmas cookies into the nutrients that make them up, but we need to be reminded that no matter what the season, the damage of excess in the cookie department still exists.

Dealing with the variety of Christmas cookies means reminding yourself of the hard work and determination you put into feeling good about yourself, and that a cookie, or a platter of them, will not override it. I prefer to make choices from the veggie tray. Even the meat and cheese platters are much better than cookie and candy trays.

Fact: the effects of gluten and sugar can mess with your hunger hormone "off" button.

This means that overconsumption and sugar go hand in hand. When people eat just one cookie, their body reacts to the simple sugar and wheat flour product by first having a difficult time digesting the cookie and inflaming the digestive tract. Then the body releases insulin to break down the glucose sugars that cause the body to be hungrier quicker despite the excess calories consumed.

I know that as lame as it might sound to eat from the meat and veggie tray, it can save your waist line the extra pounds that everyone else is resolving to lose in the first few months of the New Year.

Christmas is ONE day people!!! Even as much as I love the season, do not celebrate the entire month with food. The first of the New Year you will and always regret it. Remember that!

Putting the "B" in Christmas

Christmas time is great! Unless you do not get to spend time with the ones you love, then this time of year can be really rough.

I want to make a connection here that may not be justified or applicable to everyone:

Christmas time is a time of high stress, poor diet, and possibly depression for those living alone.

Here's a positive note to such a dark start to another Christmas blog: B vitamins in conjunction with a healthy diet can assist you through these possibly dark days. Anyone who has read this blog before understands that a healthy balance of vitamins and minerals, along with fats, proteins, and carbohydrates can maintain weight and therefore promote calmness and contentment.

B vitamins are the driving force behind the processing of key nutrients needed for the brain and body. This is in conjunction with what all of the 5 Hour Energy drink commercials have been saying. 5 Hour Energy drinks are nothing more than B vitamins, a little caffeine, and sweetener. The reason they work (besides the placebo effect) is because most people are not getting enough of the key B vitamins, specifically B6. When the body finally gets a significant dose that it has been lacking a person can feel clear headed and energized.

With the holiday season usually going hand in hand with less maintenance of the body, it is important that people either eat a diet rich in B vitamins (veggies and animal sources of protein) or supplement with a B complex vitamin.

These much needed and often forgotten B vitamins can then help the body process amino acids into neurotransmitters that the brain uses for thought process, excitement, calmness and pleasure.

Remember that the body is a complex organism and without even one of the necessary elements needed for processing and functioning, the body is not able to maintain itself. This being said, it means that when there is a lack of nutrients due to a poor diet or lack of appropriate foods (veggies, healthy fats, and animal protein sources), the body will develop mental fogginess and experience low energy levels among other possibly detrimental mental and physical effects.

So give yourself the gift of energy and heightened mental clarity this holiday season: whether you are spending time with family and friends or by yourself, consume a healthy diet rich in B vitamins to aid in managing those feelings that this time of year can provoke.

2013
New Year, Same Old You ...

I have to admit that being a person who loves the holidays, I also am glad when they are done.

I know ... I know ... I can hear my mom already saying something like "Luke, the holidays only come once a year" or "don't be such an old Grinch." To these phrases I reply with "Mom, it is not the holidays themselves, but the overabundance and how society makes you feel so obligated to partake in the celebration." To which she replies "sigh ... oh whatever."

No matter what makes up a celebration, there is usually food involved. This is how I was raised. If it is a birthday, we are having a big breakfast, some fast food for lunch, and a large dinner, followed by cake and ice cream in large quantities. After all, it is your birthday, so why not celebrate the day you were born by eating large, unhealthy quantities of food to hasten your trip to an early grave.

My point here is not the large quantities and poor quality of highly processed sugary sweet foods served up on holidays or birthdays, but the simple fact that life should not involve overindulgences.

During this New Year, or at least at the beginning of it, many people resolve to live happier and healthier lives. For some strange reason our society makes the New Year the significant milestone to start diets and change people's takes on life. I do not believe this to be a true measure: it actually sets people up for failure.

Look at the New Year using this analogy: every single day of your life so far, you have worn pants. On this specific Monday morning, however, you decide to not wear pants. Instead, you decide to wear gym shorts to work. The gym shorts are going to look and feel weird and attract attention from people no matter what. Even if a person suddenly wears shorts on a Tuesday afternoon, or Saturday night, it is still out of the norm for you and will feel weird, maybe even uncomfortable. However, after you wear shorts for a couple of weeks, people stop paying attention and you develop a new habit of wearing shorts in the morning.

My point is obviously that it is not when you start deciding to eat right, or how, but understanding that it takes time to live a healthy life, and getting used to working out and eating right will become more of a habit with time.

By starting a diet on January 1st or 2nd just because the first day is an official holiday, or even the first Monday of the year, is not going to be any easier to follow simply because of the date you chose to start. Ease into your workout and diet and find what works best for you. Advice from friends and family can be great, however remember a healthy lifestyle is YOUR choice and some techniques and workouts work best for some and not for others. Talking to a nutritionist can be useful to educate yourself about proper and recommended foods, as well as finding a workout you enjoy and will WANT to do.

January Blues

The white glittery snow from Christmas is now brown, gross, and melting. Unfortunately, the snow melts during the day then freezes again at night, leaving sheets of ice all over the sidewalk. January also marks a time for those thousands of people who signed up to run the marathon (or half marathon) to officially begin training.

OK, so we have icy outside conditions and thousands of people preparing to run a long distance outside event: what does this equate to?

EVERY TREADMILL IN EVERY GYM THROUGHOUT THE CITY IS BUSY FOR HOURS!!!!!

More importantly, January is now in the heart of the winter season. December is marked by the holiday. March offers a glimpse of springtime and possibly warmer days. January and February are the cold, sad months where people who suffer from depression or Seasonal Affective Disorder (SAD) really struggle.

Some people may not even realize they are suffering from SAD, but it is a condition where the colder winter months lead to a decline in mood. There are many different theories about why this happens, but most research shows a correlation between sunlight and vitamin D (or lack thereof) during the winter months. One of the best strategies for dealing with emotional despair is spending time outdoors in the fresh air. During the spring and summer months, relying on nature as a coping technique is far easier temperature-wise, highly effective, and can be built into a number of activities.

Unfortunately, when it is twenty degrees or colder outdoors with a slight wind-chill, few people, if any, want to go out and enjoy nature. It does not matter if you are a recovering alcoholic or a busy mom, the fact remains that you get less sun exposure, and therefore less natural Vitamin D3 during the winter season. Additionally, some people tan during the winter months, exposing themselves to UV light that actually absorbs much needed Vitamin

D, while others opt to ingest Vitamin D capsules that claim to fulfill the deficiency.

No matter how you treat the winter months, be conscious about what your body is going through. It is easy to be consumed by work, TV shows, school, children, etc. However, when your body begins to become run down, or it becomes difficult to get out of bed in the morning, you have already surpassed the early warning signs.

Pay attention to declining energy levels and/or a depressed mood. Do not ignore these symptoms as "just something you go through." Counseling is an effective tool to help many people make it through the winter months. Counseling allows clients to find why and how something affects them, and then introduces coping techniques to help during those difficult times.

Nutritionally, I continue to recommend a healthy diet rich in vegetables, animal protein sources, and unprocessed fats. Unfortunately, many veggies are not in season this time of year, but still try to keep your plate as colorful as possible. This will allow you to obtain the vitamins and minerals necessary for both body and brain functioning and will help you fight off sickness and sustain an active and positive mindset.

For now, don't slip on the ice, don't hog the treadmill, and pay attention to what your body is trying to tell you it needs.

Gluta-MINE (All Mine)!

Usually I don't discuss supplements because I truly believe that most people can obtain what they need with proper diet, exercise, and consistency. For you athletes out there, supplements can do great things to help your body maintain and recover for the next excruciating workout, as well as, for example, aid in digestion. Many people will automatically assume protein powders, creatine, pre-workouts, and some other form of energy and recovery are the first things recommended when getting involved in supplements.

Truth is, the number one thing I recommend for a sport supplement is … glutamine!

You may have heard of this white, tasteless, powdery product before and know it is labeled for recovery in certain supplements, but do you really know what it does and why you should take it?

Glutamine is the most abundant, nonessential amino acid found in the human body. The body is filled with muscle tissue whether that muscle is smooth (heart, esophagus, lungs, etc.) or striated (biceps, triceps, pecs, etc.). All muscles are made up of amino acids.

When people work out, become emotionally stressed, or have a poor diet, it becomes difficult for the body to build and maintain muscle mass. When an athlete hits the gym for an hour or longer, then we are looking at a human engine pushing past the threshold for which it was designed. The muscle fibers break down and tear (tiny tears). For your body to recover and prepare for physical exercise again, it needs to be fully healed. While the body does this naturally, it needs proper nutrition to aid the process. This is where glutamine comes in. Not that any of the twenty amino acids are more important than the other, but glutamine is used in large quantities for recovery of muscle tissue – again, smooth (digestive tract) and striated (those big biceps all guys want).

Being under constant physical stress (as is the case with athletes), glutamine helps build and maintain the muscle mass needed for their specific sports. People who are under constant emotional stress also need the recovery properties of glutamine as well, especially in the small intestine where most digestion takes place.

If we continue to ignore the daily stress we put on our bodies and continue to feed ourselves stress-inducing foods, such as Little Debbie's, processed fast foods, and so on, then we will have an obesity/health/nutritionally deprived epidemic on our hands. This is why more than 60 million people suffer from digestive problems in America among other mental and physical ailments.

Many gastroenterologists recommend glutamine to their patients to aid with digestion and recovery from GI tract problems. Proper diet and exercise is always recommended as well as consuming processed foods in moderation (which to me means completely avoid).

Omega-3 Chews—
Do Not Even Waste Your Time!

Ok, here is a lesson in Omega-3 fatty acids: these are important for brain, eyes, cardiovascular system and skin health, among many other benefits. The best source of Omega-3 is fish, which is why fish oil is so popular.

The two main fatty acids, DHA and EPA, are what you want to look for in a good Omega-3 product. Higher-end products will display how much DHA and EPA content is in their Omega-3 products. If you don't see it, don't waste your time or money on it.

Think about it this way: you go into a bar and pay $3 for a drink that is 90% water, but it is a good price. The next time you decide to pay $5 for a drink that is 80% alcohol. In all likelihood, it will take only one higher-priced drink to reach intoxication, whereas it may take three or four cheaper drinks to reach this level.

Please realize that I only use this as an analogy not as an endorsement for drinking alcohol, so do not run right out to your nearest bar!

Here's where the comparison comes in: go to a store that sells supplements and find a GOOD Omega-3 supplement. Do not rely on a cheap fish oil supplement found at your local Walmart or grocery store. While the cheaper alternatives are easier on your pocketbook, you end up getting next to none of the benefits for which you are taking fish oil in the first place.

Now, onto Omega-3 chews.

My fiancé and I were at a grocery store checkout lane the other day and I saw a package of Omega-3 chews. I read the back of the box to discover how much of a joke this product actually is. The DHA and EPA content were next to nothing and the bulk of the product was made up of sugars and cheap plant oils; in other words, candy. This product was labeled as a nutritional supplement; however it was nothing more than an expensive Starburst. It would take the equivalent of twenty chews to equal the benefits of one capsule of my Omega-3 supplement. Yep, that is a bag of Skittles or a package of licorice, just to get the Omega-3 found in higher-quality fish oil capsules.

I hate beating down a product that encourages people to eat healthy, but I strongly recommend always reading up on what you are about to buy. Do not just take something because it sways you with fancy words you hear or see advertised on TV or in magazines. Wasting time and money on this Omega-3, or any Omega-3 chew product, is just asking for an increased grocery bill with minimal benefits.

There is much more information available about the benefits of Omega-3 supplements and what to look for when buying these, which I will present at a later date. For now, though, buy a fish oil liquid capsule from a supplement store and make sure the EPA is at least 200mg and the DHA is at least 400mg. Anything lower than that and you're not reaping any benefits.

Running Season: Watch the Pounds Fall Like Leaves ... Maybe?

Something to think about here (and just stick with me as I present this idea): What if running actually increases your percentage of body fat? Not necessarily your weight overall, but your body fat?

Many people would not agree. People also likely would not spend forty-five minutes nightly on treadmills working to obtain the bodies they see on the covers of men's and women's health magazines.

You probably do not want to hear this, but the truth is that bouts of steadily paced cardiovascular activity can actually trigger fat storage rather than fat burning in the body!

99.99% of a human's genetic code is established before birth. Because the body is designed to maintain life, when faced with a long bout of endurance it is more efficient for the body's lifesaving function to store fat and burn muscle rather than the other way around.

Unfortunately, when many people begin weight-loss programs, running is almost always incorporated. This activity will help burn more calories, that's for sure, but if muscle stimulation is ignored then the weight-loss program goals will not be fully met. Muscles actually burn more calories the remaining twenty-three hours of a day than one hour of cardio can burn. In my experience, weight / interval training has always been far more effective than running for long periods of time. An added bonus is that interval/weight training also can be done in a shorter amount of time.

No, not every person who runs is fat, and regular runners usually are pretty thin, appearance wise, however many have a higher percentage of body fat and less muscle so they don't look "bulky." I am for the most part referring to those seasonal runners who sign up to run occasional marathons or half marathons. In most cases, people begin to train excessively, causing the body to burn muscle and store fat.

Because muscle serves as extra weight, to maintain itself during long runs the body will begin to digest muscle tissue for energy. This is very inefficient and hard on the body because when the body needs glucose it is forced to break down the amino acids necessary to maintain and build muscle. This process is called gluconeogenesis. So the next time you decide to sign up for a half marathon with the goal of losing weight, remember you may be doing more damage to your metabolic-increasing muscle tissue than if you incorporated weight training or a form of high intensity interval training into your workout.

Muscle is fat's worst enemy, and maintaining more muscle will lead to greater energy and overall satisfaction. Overall than, dare I say, a skinny, muscle-deprived, runner's body.

One last tip here for all seasonal runners: you do not need to increase your carbohydrate intake for half marathons, 5k, or 10k races that occur every other weekend. In fact, the body can efficiently store up to five hundred grams of carbohydrates in the body, which is approximately enough to run 10 miles without needing extra energy. Instead, eat a diet rich in vegetables, lean meats, and fats obtained from nuts, fish, or unrefined oils. These EFFICIENT foods will give you the energy needed for a good run or outdoor activity. Carbohydrates are quick energy sources, but will only store as fat. Again, if you just got done running, or even if you won't run unless chased, use fats and proteins as your energy and food source rather than bread, rice, and fruits.

Sweeteners ... Not Natural, But Can Be a Big Help to Maintaining a Healthy Diet

Usually I recommend eating natural, unaltered foods full of nutrients the body needs for efficient digestion and absorption.

When it comes to stressful days, celebrations, or just wanting something sweet, artificially-sweetened products (Splenda, aspartame, Stevia, saccharine, erythritol) can allow some wiggle room and can satisfy cravings.

Enough people put down artificial sweeteners that I would like to express some of their benefits. The positive aspects of artificially sweetened products, such as diet soda, sugar-free gum, sugar-free candy, no sugar added ice cream, or other sweetened products, can actually outweigh the negative effects when looking at the big picture of life.

An artificial sweetener is a chemical that binds to the sweet receptors of the tongue in such a fashion that the signals it sends to the brain mimic that of actual sugar. Better yet, artificial sweeteners do not convert to glucose in the blood stream and therefore do not force the body to raise blood sugar levels. They also help avoid fat storage, sugar crashes, and the release of dopamine that is caused from eating sugar and products that contain high fructose corn syrup.

Unfortunately, as a society we have set ourselves up for failure since birth. The younger the generation, the more likely they are to become obese and/or develop new previously-unheard-of or never-encountered diseases even to my generation (children born in the 80s). Americans have become increasingly overindulgent and over-consume increasingly sweeter products. Some people are never satisfied and feel that sweet foods are their only pleasure in life, so they eat them. In conjunction with this shifting perception, the more sugar is consumed, the more sugar is craved, leading to a person having higher body fat and a higher risk of cardiovascular disease.

In the current Diagnostic and Statistical Manual of Mental Disorders (aka the Bible for diagnosing mental health), Binge Eating Disorder may be effecting many people who aren't even aware they are suffering from a life-destroying problem.

The point here is that this increasingly sweet and sedentary world in which we are living is resulting in calories and sugar intake going up while activity and nutrition continue to decrease. Many clients with whom I talk about sugar do not even understand that high fructose corn syrup and sugar, in its many forms, can be the culprit behind a sudden weight gain, lack of energy, difficulty in concentration, or cravings that can actually cause a person to sleepwalk and consume excessive calories without even noticing. All of these symptoms stem from insulin-raising, sugar-containing products.

For healthy, satisfying recipes that use less sugar, I recommend websites that cater to the needs of diabetics. However, with knowledge, you can go into any recipe, replace some things, and make it to your needs and enjoyment.

I do not recommend artificially sweetened products on a daily basis. Save these for times when something sweet is absolutely necessary. (Think "in case of emergency break glass" type situations.)

Tell Those Cravings To Go To Bed!

In this day and age, it appears that people are busier, getting less sleep, and are more stressed than previous generations. While technology is making the world a seemingly easier place to live, its conveniences and advances also make it very difficult to shut off electronics and to get restorative sleep.

Here is a strong correlation: when sleep declines, body fat increases!

Think about it. People are sleeping less now than ever before and as active as people supposedly are during these extra wakeful hours, this is actually proving a fallacy: people are gaining, not losing weight.

Let's say that there is a night you are up late doing homework, focusing on a project for work, out with friends, or even gaming. Staying up later than your normal bedtime throws off your usual sleep pattern to the point where you are overly tired the next day. When someone is tired, nutritionally they tend to crave higher caloric, processed foods containing sugar, salt, and minimal nutrients.

Think energy drinks, chips, cookies, and coffee drinks chock-full of sugar and hydrogenated oils.

High calorie, processed foods are destroying the late night adventurer and putting healthy broccoli and fish on the back burner. My hope is that by bringing this to light people will be more aware of their "cravings" and why they truly occur. Counselors call this mindfulness!

The stress hormone cortisol is one that will continue to be increasingly relevant to a tech-addicted society. When a body is overtaxed, up late, doesn't get enough sleep, and experiences stress (coupled with crappy foods), cortisol is released, forcing the body to store body fat. It also destabilizes blood sugar levels, increases cravings for sugary and salty, processed foods, lowers energy levels, decreases positive moods, increases agitation, decreases muscle tissue, and leaves one feeling constantly dissatisfied.

One simple solution is to stop staying up so late. You have to decide if getting that extra gaming in, homework done, work project completed, or a little more time with friends is worth destroying your body in the long run. I know what my answer would be!

Staying up late or getting only a few hours less of sleep a night makes you think about all of the foods that bring immediate pleasure, because, after all, you are tired and weak. Staying up late actually decreases testosterone in men and fatigues the body to where the recovery and rebuilding of muscle structure is no longer the body's primary function. The body is now overtaken by its primal need to exist through storing fat. Think about it. Fruit and veggie stands aren't open all night for the reason that people want processed salt and sugar in its many forms at that hour.

While socially it may be acceptable to stay up late, drink sugary drinks, and eat fast food before bed, it is also the "western culture" to gain weight. While many people in America may become obese for any number of reasons, why add one more to the list? Get some rest and allow the next day to be a healthy, relaxed one.

Making the Connection between Pain and Mental Health ... a Plug for Mental Health Counseling

While the content of this blog is 98% nutrition, health, and working out, today I wanted to discuss a topic to inspire readers to attempt new ways to fix old problems.

Think of how you might feel if you had chronic back problems: every day the area surrounding your back muscles is inflamed leading to restricted movement, pain, and discomfort. Now, when you go to your doctor he diagnoses you with some sort of degenerative discs, muscle spasms, or some medical term I am not qualified to understand right now. His answer is to prescribe rest and a pain medication. So you take his advice, get the prescription filled, go home, and now face the added stress of a serious, diagnosed problem with your back. Have you ever considered that the pain in your back was actually all in your head?

You may become upset with me, tune me out, or stop reading altogether. Please consider that I am not asking you to change everything you believe, including that your physical pain isn't real. Regardless of whether pain is radiating due to inflammation from the actual site, it is the brain that interprets the signal as pain and it is definitely real. This pain needs to be dealt with to improve your quality of life.

Just remember that doctors treat symptoms. When you go in with chronic backaches the recommended treatment will likely consist of pain medications and relaxation. For longer term benefits you could go to a chiropractor who would adjust and realign your spinal cord which would then realign your muscles and therefore improve posture and even possibly resolve stomach problems.

What if instead of going to a medical doctor to get examined and prescribed something temporarily you went to a mental health counselor who helped resolve issues in your subconscious mind? The brain could stop dealing with hidden or suppressed emotions and therefore possibly stop creating psychosomatic symptoms that are depicted as pain and very real to you, the client.

Don't get me wrong: there are definitely ailments that need to be handled by a medical doctor, surgeon, or specialist. However, there are also chronic aches and pains that seem to correlate with mental health issues, such as depression and anxiety. No amount of medication can release what has built up or been suppressed in the subconscious mind over time.

For some people maybe even a placebo-like effect would occur where just the thought of treatment by a doctor, pain meds, or other specialist works as an identifiable fixer. The general population does not really care what "fixes" them as long as they feel better. The truth is that with any medication and/or surgery there are both resulting short and long-term side effects. Seeing a mental health counselor comes with no side effects and the client benefits from becoming more independent through working out their own problems rather than relying on a temporary solution.

Let's revisit the example of the gentleman with a chronic back problem who is finally fed up with the pain and decides to see a mental health counselor to help deal with the extra stress of chronic pain. During the first session, the mental health counselor realizes there are some anger issues the gentleman has never addressed. The client feels that he cannot openly share or express his anger because he has learned to suppress it and move on. Many families find it unacceptable to express or process anger and therefore discourage it.

All the years of suppressing anger has now manifested itself in physical pain for this client.

After a few weeks of anger management, the client learns coping techniques that help him effectively deal with his anger. Eventually, his back problems may even disappear. When the mind is allowed to relax and is given tools for handling stressful situations, the body also adjusts, relaxes, and begins handling stressful situations more efficiently.

The disease of alcoholism is a good example of this.

In many cases people drink to cope with stressful, tough times. Maybe they experienced crappy childhoods, their work sucks, or their spouse is difficult. Whatever the reason, that person now has a physiological drive to drink alcohol. Furthermore, an addiction also creates withdrawal when there is no alcohol in the person's system. Well, let's make the connection. Addiction is a disease initiated by not being able to manage your own mental discomfort. A similar condition of mental anguish is caused by years of suppressed anger or anxiety. The brain doesn't know how to handle these stressors.

Think how you could save money, time, and possible side effects by looking internally at your own stressors, anger level, or any past unresolved issues.

What Keeps the Motivation?

If I could sit here and type relevant, interesting information that would convince people they need to consume more fish, drink less soda, and get more sleep at night I would be rich. If it were only that easy – but it's not.

Truth be told (and I think my nutrition clients understand this), when times get tough, the most difficult thing in the world, it seems, is to maintain a healthy diet.

It's funny because when the world becomes stressful, you are working double shifts, or there is an illness or death in the family, it is considered socially acceptable to comfort oneself with highly processed, sugar-rich foods. Think back to a funeral you may have attended. Remember the lunch afterwards? I doubt it consisted of chicken breasts. Instead, I am guessing there were little sandwiches and pastries for dessert.

During stressful times in life, we should be consuming healthy, nutrient-rich foods to help reduce the emotional fluctuations that can occur with blood sugar spikes and crashes.

Yet I cannot deny that a doughnut, cherry turnover, or, at my house, German chocolate cake, tastes better than broccoli ever could, but that feeling of pleasure is so short-lived that at some point you have to ask yourself: what is the point? We consume sugary, fatty treats to deal with stress because, for a short while, it works. It works because of the dopamine that is released when we consume sugar or products that quickly convert to sugar in the body, such as breads, pastas, rice, and other processed foods.

Motivation needs to remain high when you are trying to get control over food instead of letting food control you. When it is Thursday and a coworker brings doughnuts to work and you forgot your breakfast, it is up to you and your level of motivation to find an alternative to giving in to the doughnut because obviously it does not have the same nutritional content as your Greek yogurt and blueberries.

Or how about this scenario: it is Saturday night and you have had a few drinks with your friends and the bars are closing. While everybody suggests going to IHOP for a stack of pancakes, you need to opt for the veggie omelet, even though your state of impulsiveness and lack of caution to whim tells you otherwise.

These little but constant decisions are what separate fit and healthy people from those envious out-of-shape ones. The right decision has to be made consistently, and, unfortunately, seeing a counselor, nutritionist, or doctor cannot help you maintain motivation. While there are tips and tricks to help in times of extreme craving, such as some alternative recipes I give my clients, their motivation level is what helps some choose healthy options over poor, but good-tasting options.

Consistency leads to satisfaction in life and the body prefers this state of consistency! Inconsistency leads to stress, anxiety, and a level of unknowing which can lead to imbalances in the body and, in extreme cases, mental disorders.

Think about it this way: if I wanted a college degree I would not show up to a class every so often, take a few tests, stop for a while, then start up and stop over and over again. That would not make sense and it would take me many years to get a degree that way. The same goes with weight loss, or at least gaining a sense of control over food cravings and the desire to constantly eat poorly. It takes eating healthy every day, at every meal, and being consistent with workouts. Even for those who "fall off the wagon" nutritionally, they can hop right back on, getting their mindset back to an imperfect and forgiving world rather than a rigid black and white one.

Knowledge is something that can help people through difficult times of deciding what to eat. For the most part, my nutrition clients have a general understanding of what types of foods (as opposed to specifics) to eat early on. This means that they usually know a doughnut is not a good option for breakfast, but they do not always know why. This is where knowledge can help ingrain the idea that a doughnut is sugar, fat and bread, none of which are beneficial for the body. Therefore a doughnut is not a good choice.

In summary: life is a marathon, not a sprint, and eating healthy should be treated as such. However, do not jump right into asparagus and boiled chicken breasts at every meal. Get a sense over time of what you like and what works best for you. Seeing a nutritional counselor, such as myself, can help clients gain a better understanding, keep them accountable for their choices, and keep their progress on track.

ADD Versus Sugar High

When a person consumes sugar, or any food that quickly converts to sugar in the blood stream (AKA blood glucose), the body automatically releases the hormone insulin in an attempt to remove sugar from the blood before it becomes toxic.

When glucose is pulled from the blood stream and distributed to other body parts or the brain, the body also releases adrenaline, the same substance that is released when a person is skydiving from a plane or driving a race car.

Now think about a child's typical cafeteria meal. I had the opportunity a few years back to work in a middle school and observe a pre-teenage group of students as they chose what they wanted for lunch. Every single option contained bread, in high amounts, usually pasta, breaded meats, sandwiches, tortillas, and, of course, dessert!

These kids were exposed to enough carbohydrates to fuel them through running a full marathon, yet after lunch they were expected to sit quietly for a few more hours of learning. Many kids are diagnosed with inattentiveness, over-activity, impulsivity, or a combination leading to the diagnosis of (drum roll) ... Attention Deficit Hyperactivity Disorder (ADHD),simply because they were first loaded up with carbohydrates and then told to sit and pay attention to the teacher discussing world geography ... yawn!

Of course, not every child responds as negatively to carbohydrates as may be indicated here. However, why would we even risk putting a child on ADHD medicine because they have a hard time sitting still in class due to possible dietary problems? Adrenaline that is released in children usually does not even reach its peak until approximately an hour after consumption of a simple, carbohydrate-rich meal. This means kids are at risk of "undesirable behaviors" in the afternoon, or immediately after breakfast in some schools because of all the sugar they consume.

Question: "but doesn't everything we eat turn into sugar in the body anyway, so why does it matter if the food is carbohydrates, fats, or proteins?"

Answer: Your body has three hormones that are involved in raising its blood sugar level, and only one that helps lower it. Therefore, our bodies are more adapted to maintaining stable blood sugars than continuously lowering the blood sugar level. However, do not mistakenly compare and equate how the body can hormonally raise its own blood sugar level with consuming sugar in copious amounts; they are not the same. These occur in much different ways. All carbohydrates turn to sugar in the blood, but how quickly this reaction occurs depends on the amount and type of carbohydrate that is consumed. The simpler the sugar, the quicker the reaction, the more adrenaline is released.

Remember: lowering the amount of carbohydrates children consume, or, at least changing the carbohydrate source, allows the body to react more positively and calmly to the foods that are eaten. Stay away from bread products, any products containing fructose and sucrose, and just avoid large quantities of carbohydrates altogether. (Granola is horrible.)

So let us all agree to at least give the youth of our nation a chance by feeding them properly. Meals should include a good animal protein source, vegetables, a healthy fat source, and a small amount of a nutrient-rich carbohydrate source such as quinoa, yams, vegetables, or oatmeal just to name a few. While this may increase the price of meals, it will ultimately lower expensive pharmacy and medical bills that are paid to keep our youth sitting still in class.

Nutritional Counseling Can Shine a Light on a Dark Topic

I wish I could tell you that losing weight or getting control over food was as easy as eat this, not that. It is not. I wish I could give advice on eating a lettuce wrap instead of using bread for a sandwich or wrap, but that does not taste as good. I wish that chocolate, doughnuts, cakes, ice cream, candy, and alcohol were not as pleasurable, but they are.

The old way of looking at losing weight or gaining control over food was called dieting. I hate the word "dieting" because, to me, it means temporary. For example, whenever people ask me about a "diet" I might recommend, I really have a hard time not responding that when weight is lost via a restrictive diet, when the diet is no longer followed, the weight will come right back. Anybody can do something for a short amount of time, such as follow a diet, but it is those people who make life changes and decide they want to live healthy lives who end up keeping off the excess weight. Research shows that most dieters put the weight back on within 12 months. It is interesting to me how many of my clients struggle, not necessarily with weight loss, but with the constant pleasure of food and guilt of over consumption twenty-four hours a day.

"Why do we crave food?"

I remind my clients that food is pleasurable. Food is the original drug! Companies have refined food into processed junk that, in my opinion, is more addictive and detrimental than any drug or alcohol addiction. When high-fructose corn syrup and wheat gluten touches your lips, dopamine is quickly released in the brain, creating a sensation of pleasure experienced simply by eating a floury, sugary, deep-fat-fried treat (like doughnuts for example). Doughnuts are legal, cheap, available, and in often cases highly encouraged, leading to over consumption. So you tell me what is one of the hardest addictions to break?

I say food addiction.

Sometimes, pleasurable responses from food can be a good thing leading us to remember fond, comforting memories; however, when a person starts to rely more steadily on that pleasure then we start to have issues. Unfortunately, I notice a lot of people addicted to processed foods and they do not even know it until they are told to watch their weight or triglyceride levels by the doctor. It is then that they realize those few doughnuts in the morning could be killing them. By then the addiction has taken over, and with little thought the mouth is already salivating over that rich, flaky texture of a doughnut, cinnamon roll, or fill in the gap with your favorite pleasure:_____.

Treatment with me involves weekly sessions discussing the past week's successes and failures along with future roadblocks to success. Food journals show a pattern so clients can begin to identify their emotional triggers, eating patterns, and to get a Polaroid snapshot of what their typical diet looks like. I recommend this activity for anybody who struggles with food management. As with any mental health concern or potential addiction, the problem needs to be treated where it all starts: the brain. Identifying negative thought processes can prevent negative, self-destructive decisions to overeat and can avoid the remorse that follows.

Going to a Resort, Wedding Trippin!

Recently, I was lucky enough to marry my best friend on the beach at a resort in Cabo San Lucas, Mexico. I will start off by saying that the weather down there in the middle of May is simply amazing, the people are so nice, and the all-inclusive resort package honestly could have killed me!

People who read my blog, or at least those who know me, understand that at times I can shut off reasoning and enjoy the indulgences of life. Trust me, there have been instances of me eating an entire large pizza followed by a half gallon of ice cream. I'm not proud of it, but there it is. Even this past Cinco de Mayo I entered and beat a food challenge that involved downing five enchiladas and a large taco within 10 minutes. I got a free shirt! It was pretty amazing!

So, as you can see, periodically letting food dominate me is no big deal, however doing this for seven days and six nights, including all of the free slushy multicolored (SUGAR FILLED) drinks I want is way beyond what I can handle. I might not have literally died, but I would have lost a couple of years of life due to eating as much of what I wanted. Restraint was honestly my best friend for many reasons, but the main reason is because I wanted to enjoy Mexico and actually do things instead of just lying around all day feeling like crap.

This was a challenge too. I mean as soon as we stepped foot off the airplane the cab driver offered us mixed drinks. Then, on the way to the resort we were offered a beer. When we checked in, a cocktail waitress gave us drinks. An all-day buffet served up fried food, pizzas, sweets, and ice cream. In the room there was booze along with a minibar full of sugary sodas. Again, I can clearly overindulge, but then usually I am shut down and go home and sleep because I'm so miserable. Honestly, fatty foods affect me so much that I know my day is ruined once I've consumed them. Everything from my mood, motivation, and energy levels just take a dive. I want to do nothing more than eat more food or lay around waiting to eat more food.

The first few days I indulged in the buffet's fatty foods. I even consumed many of those colorful drinks (which contain hardly any alcohol, but a ton of calories). After a few days, the food got old and the drinks weren't exciting anymore: that is when I really began to enjoy the trip. At dinner I would still indulge in a little fancy dessert, but for the most part during the day I ate vegetables, meat, and as healthy of fat sources as I could find. Remember: these healthy foods cost more than breaded/fried foods and are harder to reheat; therefore breaded/fried foods were more readily available than any grouper or salmon filet.

Once your entertainment of the day shifts from food to the actual reason you're on vacation, then you can really start living. I enjoyed the simple parts of the trip: the weather, reading by the pool, family, friends, and just being able to relax. My overall satisfaction level went up once I stopped worrying about all of the food I was going to eat and started focusing on what was most important: the wedding!

Once back home, I enjoyed a large egg white and spinach omelet. I enjoyed raw unsalted almonds. I also missed my scoop of natural peanut butter combined with protein powder and formed into what I call a peanut butter cookie. Needless to say after the vacation, I needed to get a vacation from processed foods!

S'more What? You're Killin' Me Smalls!

Remember that movie *The Sandlot*? Of course you do. It was an amazing tale of a boy who was new to town and his journey to make friends. Eventually there are some baseball games, some hijinks, and a large dog at the end that teaches all the boys a lesson: not to judge a book by its cover!

Great Story!

I want to elaborate on what I saw during the movie. I noticed a bunch of adolescent boys being active, playing sports, going to the pool, and staying out of the house most of the day. Now, I am in no way saying that what happens in this movie is real life anymore, however what I am trying to point out on this warm day is that the sooner youth get outdoors, the sooner they establish healthy habits.

Facts:

- Vitamin D is absorbed best in its natural form of D3 from sunlight.
- The more active a person, the more neurotransmitters are released to lower the likelihood of depression.
- Being outdoors can inspire creativity and build an appreciation for nature, thereby encouraging people to respect and preserve it.
- Even just walking outdoors can burn 3-4 times as many calories as sitting indoors watching TV, playing video games, etc.

Some of these benefits are common sense, yet we still ignore and avoid them. I know that on those hot summer days when it reaches one hundred and ten degrees, I probably will not be spending too much time outdoors myself, no matter what I am wearing (after all, there is a limit to how low you can go). I much prefer the coldness of winter anyway.

I notice that adolescents do not spend time outside like previous generations did. Youth seem to take much for granted: things like air conditioning, video games, movies, the internet, texting, Tweeting, Skype, even reading books indoors is keeping them too comfortable. It seems that as new generations come along, the level of laziness rises. One day we will all end up on a spaceship sitting in our mobile chairs watching shopping networks, like in the Pixar movie, *WALL-E*.

While I don't want to let my anxious, often negative view of the world consume my thoughts, as far as good nutrition and healthy living are concerned, we absolutely have got to be more active outdoors. Get dirty, scrape your knees, make up some games, just shut the TV off (or unplug it and test your kids by making sure it is still cool once you get home like my mom used to do).

It is difficult to compete with the immediate pleasure of video games such as *Halo* or *Gears of War*, but we have done this to ourselves. I know that if your child goes back to school the next year with a healthy tan and lean muscle mass from running and playing all summer (not to mention the social skills and friendships acquired), he will be more confident and less likely to resort to negative means of obtaining attention.

Adolescent attention spans are decreasing due in part to the immediate stimulation of iPads, iPhones, and overly processed, cheap, and readily available sugar sources. When children are healthier as a result of stimulating physical activity, they also are more likely to possess higher self-esteem and command more positive attention from others as opposed to having to resort to acting out to attract any kind of attention at all.

To summarize with a scene from *The Sandlot:* there is a point in the movie where they are making s'mores up in a treehouse, looking out for the dog next door. It was always funny to me that nobody really cared about the s'mores more than the "overweight" catcher. Watching that part, for some reason, really made a s'more sound really good, but I didn't want to be the "overweight" kid, so I would always act like I could have cared less about s'mores.

P.S. I WAS that overweight child! :)

The Truth about Those Supplement Claims …

Supplements are great for everyone, um … supplements are great. OK, one more time, supplements are … well, actually it is hard to categorize supplements as all good or all bad, or sometimes anything.

I have taken, worked around, sold, recommended and not recommended various supplements in my life. On one end of the spectrum I was that scrawny 16–year-old boy looking at *Muscle and Fitness* magazine, reading about the bodybuilders and what "supplements" they took. I knew that when I was old enough and had money I could take those supplements and get BIG too. On the other end I was the "BIG" guy who was now recommending that people take what I take. I was scraping up money while in college at age seventeen to keep taking my protein powder and pre-workout supplements that I knew I NEEDED. I did this up until I found myself working multiple jobs and spending hundreds of dollars a month on various supplements that I continued to convince myself I NEEDED. I am not saying they did not work, or that they did not serve their purpose at the time, but I wonder what quality food I could have bought with the same money I spent on supplements and what type of results I would have had by doing that.

Enough about me: this post is to help people better understand supplements and why they are such a large industry raking in anywhere from $60-70 billion in annual sales and employing more than 450,000 people. That is great for the economy, but is every cent of that money actually going towards something, or is that $70 billion spent on hope and nothing more?

The funny thing is that if I went over every supplement and ingredient, explained each one's supposed effect on the body, but then revealed the AMOUNT actually needed to be shown effective, it would really help people understand why supplement companies can claim what they claim without technically lying. It also would take a person years to analyze the thousands of pages of data and information. Believe it or not, I am not going to do that here. No, I would rather people understand that for 99% of the population supplements really have no effect.

Proper nutrition, exercise, sleep, and lowered stress: these are things that people can do for themselves that have a much larger impact on how they look, feel, and act. These actions have more impact than any supplement ever could. The placebo effect is huge, and not just in the supplement industry, but in the pharmaceutical industry as well. I wrote an earlier post about the importance of the mind-body connection in how a person responds to pain and how positivity has been shown to increase a person's pain tolerance and speed up recovery time. Mind you, these were people with injuries who sought counseling to help deal with underlying anxiety, depression, and traumas. So can you imagine how people may respond to a physical pill or powder that CLAIMS to make you run faster, jump higher, even look better? The placebo effect has a person even before they buy the product.

I sold supplements for more than two years and I even convinced myself that some of the lower quality products we never recommended were still worth the money because their claims were so bold. Ah, but as I described earlier, all a supplement has to do is put an ingredient into a product and it can then claim all of the benefits associated with that ingredient, even if you need ten times the amount given to get results.

For example: let's say that research has shown that six grams of fish oil increases focus and thinking ability and decreases the chances of having Alzheimer's disease. Ok, so if I develop a product and put fifty milligrams of fish oil in my supplement, I can now claim that this product will make you smarter! Yeah, it is a pretty bold claim, but not completely untrue. Never mind that the researched amount is 120 times more than what is in my supplement, and who knows how long the person has to take fish oil to notice increased focus and thinking ability. I could even bulk up my supplement by adding freeze-dried fruits and then claim things like strong enough antioxidant amounts in my supplement to actually kill cancer cells. No, you do not kill cancer; however, you may possibly be able to reduce its spread and severity with antioxidants found in whole natural foods – but this is not a revolutionary thing. Remember, the nutrients in whole foods are more effectively absorbed in proper quantities than any supplement.

Another factor to consider when looking at supplements is the process used to obtain a specific nutrient because nutrients do not last very long once the organism is no longer alive. Even whole foods contain phytonutrients with a very short shelf life. Antioxidants and vitamins quickly leach out of food. For example, cooking can significantly reduce the nutrient content of foods. So I can only imagine how processed and packaged protein powders, vitamins, and sports enhancing supplements may contain very little nutritional or health-related value.

Supplements cannot undo what you have been genetically given no matter how colorful the package or how bold the claim. So understand that there are limits to what your body is able to do athletically or health-wise, BUT do not give in or give up: build upon YOUR strengths.

The Truth about Those Supplement Claims … (part 2)

Creatine, glutamine, multivitamins, protein powders, fish oils, Tryptophan, GABA are all supplements I currently take. Now, according to my previous post it is not recommended or necessary to take supplements because:

A. It is impossible to undo genetics.
B. In many situations the supplement may be devoid of any actual benefit.
C. The vitamin and mineral content found in supplements are insignificant to produce any benefit.

Even though I know that supplements really do not help grow muscles, expand muscle tissue, or impact how muscles react during workouts, I continue to take a core amount of supplements to help the 5% of my body that can use these benefits. When putting my body through high amounts of stress, such as what occurs with periods of long, intense running, lifting, or a combination of aerobic and anaerobic activity, my body uses up key nutrients. Deficiencies in certain nutrients then lead the body to pull those nutrients from existing tissue.

For example, when the body doesn't get enough protein, or goes too long with a nitrogen imbalance (the only nutrient to release nitrogen is protein), it begins to break down its own muscle tissue to get the nitrogen needed for recovery. See, the body will always win out when it needs something regardless of our goal to burn fat. If, however, before the workout a person consumes a protein or protein supplement (preferably from an animal source such as whey, Casein, egg whites, red meat, but not soy), the body now has a ready amount of all essential amino acids and can release nitrogen into the blood stream. In turn, this will preserve muscles during an intense workout and allow the body to burn fat for energy.

Yes, there are benefits to taking supplements. I just want to emphasize to not go "over the top" with them. Do not rely solely on supplements to do the job for you. You are the one who has to work out, eat nutrient rich foods, and stay away from toxins, sugars, and unhealthy fats. In the long run, this will have a larger impact than any supplement ever could. Being honest here, I know that some supplements I take are not NEEDED, however – placebo or not – I can notice benefits, in small amounts. I believe that the little help I get from my supplements is noticeable. Sometimes with my busy schedule I do not have the opportunity to get all my nutrients from the food I eat alone, and the boost a concentrated supplement can provide is just enough.

So even though the previous post seemed to put a negative spin on supplements, I really just want consumers to understand the benefits and formulation differences among supplements and that not all supplements are credible or effective. Do your own research; decide on your own budget; and if you find something that works for you, no matter if it is a placebo or the real deal, try it out for a while. Just be critical when reading supplement labels as information can be presented in a misleading way. Also, if you find something that works for you, stick with it. Trust me: the grass is not always greener.

Take a little time to look up the active ingredient in the supplement and see if there are any actual benefits. Also look at how many you may need to take to obtain those benefits. This is particularly important where weight loss pills are concerned (which I do not recommend) because those are some of the largest grossing products in the supplement world and some have been known to make outrageous, even dangerous claims!

However, we will go ahead and save that topic for another day.

Hormones, Nutrition and PMS: Ladies (and Gents) Listen Up!

Hormone imbalances can cause a wide range of problems including:

- Premenstrual Syndrome (PMS)
- Infertility
- Postpartum depression
- Menopause and peri-menopause
- Female sexual dysfunction
- Testosterone deficiency
- Osteoporosis
- Chronic fatigue
- Fibromyalgia
- Endometriosis
- Andropause (male menopause)
- Hypothyroidism and hyperthyroidism
- Hypoadrenalism

So, with that in mind, let's get started. While this is of particular interest to ladies, it also can affect guys too.

While I am not a doctor, unlike many doctors I do know something about nutrition and how it works to improve many health issues, including hormonal problems experienced by many women. First and foremost, get rid of processed foods and replace them with real, nutrient- rich foods. This will start to even out the hormonal imbalances that are becoming more prevalent. The key is knowing which diet and specific nutrients will work for you and your specific problem. While most hormonal imbalances usually occur later in life, it is not unusual to experience them at any age especially when caused by physiological disorders. As you may have guessed, weight gain and water retention are just a couple of the frustrating life issues that go hand in hand with imbalanced hormones.

Some nutritional recommendations are:

1. Eat regular meals 5-6 times throughout the day to maintain blood sugar levels. Your metabolism peaks at noon, so consuming most of your calories at night can lead to excessive weight gain and low blood sugar throughout the following morning.
2. Consume a healthy protein source with each meal, usually nothing above 20-25 grams per meal (fish, meat, eggs, even a protein supplement). Anything above 20-25 grams can actually cause the body to react as if carbohydrates were ingested.
3. Lower your intake of carbohydrates. Insulin is released when carbohydrates are consumed, and because insulin is itself a hormone, its constant spiking and crashing can throw off other hormones directly affecting PMS.
4. Lower/eliminate your grain intake (whole wheat, flour, breads, and crackers, for example). If it contains grain stay away. The imbalances caused by gluten have been researched and shown to have a negative effect on overall health.
5. Eat more veggies. Veggies contain many nutrients that the body physically craves due to necessity. When the body does not receive needed nutrients, the brain sends out a chemical response known as a craving to satisfy this need (think cravings related to a woman's monthly menstrual cycle and to pregnancy — both relate to hormonal imbalances).
6. Eat foods rich in antioxidants. Antioxidants protect the body from oxidation (duh, it's in the name) and are linked to the reduction of cancer through elimination of free radicals.

Blood work is needed to fully determine the nutrients/hormones a person is either deficient in or has an excess of, both of which can lead to an imbalance. Much research I have read on hormone imbalance recommends diets that I have discussed on this blog anyway, which is just another reason why a nutrient-rich diet low in processed foods can significantly help people get back to the simple pleasures of life and good health.

Cholesterol starts the process of developing hormones, but if healthy cholesterol is not consumed (such as that found in high carbohydrate, low fat diets) then we have a problem. The body needs cholesterol, but when a diet is lacking in it, the body will use its own, which in turn raises cholesterol levels in the bloodstream (also accounting for why getting a cholesterol test after eating a high carbohydrate meal as opposed to a low carb, high fat meal could result in higher cholesterol levels). It also takes nutrients to convert cholesterol into pregnenolone, the hormone that is the starting point for most hormone development (for just one example). Referring back to the dietary recommendations I mentioned earlier will help the body properly convert food into healthy hormones and maintain a balance in the body.

What's Wrong with Sugar Free?

Skinny Girl margaritas, mojitos, and martinis, which depict a skinny little girl on their labels, contain less sugar and fewer calories than regular, sugar-filled alcoholic drinks. While alcohol isn't good in the first place, combining it with high fructose corn syrup can be one of the worst combinations since people started mixing cough syrup and Sprite. (The codeine in cough syrup gets people high, but kills more brain cells and deteriorates muscle response time at such a rapid rate that it is truly one of the worst, most lethal combinations ever). So what's wrong with sugar free alcoholic drinks? Mostly the stereotype associated with people who order them. If you go to the bar and order a vodka and sugar-free Red Bull it must be for your girlfriend, or wife, right? Nope, it is actually mine!

Guys are naturally assumed to be dark beer and full sugar soda drinkers, and consumers of the biggest, beefiest hamburgers a restaurant has to offer. The females however get dainty drinks full of color and a salad. For example: a couple comes into a restaurant and part of their order includes a salad. The waiter more than likely will assume it is for the woman, but, no, it is the man's (this story was and continues to be true in my life). So, what is the big deal if I like my greens and dressing on the side along with some chicken or salmon? Why is it considered so out of the realm of possibility that the leaner meal is mine?

I could discuss the benefits of eating healthy and even discuss point-by-point how leaner meals actually lead to men growing bigger and stronger than greasy hamburgers, but why waste my breath when anybody who has a sliver of knowledge (or has been reading this blog up until now) knows. Greasy, processed, sugar-filled, and trans-fat-containing foods can actually decrease testosterone levels and raise estrogen levels to the point where those man boobs actually start to form into real boobs. Research has shown that eating nutrient rich foods, lower processed fats, and lower amounts of sugar and soy can actually raise testosterone levels in males. Increased muscle mass and density, lower body fat, healthier fat distribution, and higher amounts of energy actually lead to what we stereotypically define as masculinity.

Ok, now here we are again at the bar ordering a drink after working out six days this week, working two jobs, and keeping the significant other happy. We want to relax a little bit, but not throw away all of the progress in lean muscle mass tissue that has been made the entire last week. So what to order? I choose an alcohol that is low on the glycemic index (vodka) and combine it with either water (always safe) or attempt a diet soda mixture (not always safe). A few of these puppies and you feel good enough to relax without the sugar high associated with more colorful drinks.

Now, if you're at home and want a martini, mojito, or margarita then there is nothing wrong with a low-sugar/sugar-free option to continue in the right direction of healthy choices. Again, speaking from a male point of view, I would probably only make these drinks at home because drinking these stereotypically feminine drinks in public could take my masculine persona down a couple notches, much like the pink sugar-free *Rockstar* drink which I accidentally bought and noticed it came with a straw on the side.

Nutritionally, sugar-free drinks combined with alcohol will help keep those abdominal muscles in picture-perfect shape more so than colorful, sugar-filled drinks. As a male, experiment with some of the sugar-free mixes and *Skinny Girl* drinks – just keep the bottle hidden when serving your friends unless you are brave enough to take the "girlie" drink comments that are bound to come your way. Hey, blame society for this one folks, not me.

Melatonin, the Original Antidepressant!

Melatonin is produced by UV rays. The pineal gland in the brain converts light into melatonin that starts a chain reaction of events in the body which results in the release of growth hormone, cortisol, and DHEA. All of these hormones serve important functions related to mood and thought regulation. The pituitary gland controls all sexual desires and functions by releasing hormones that lead to the production of testosterone in men and estrogen in women.

In a previous post I discussed hormone imbalances and what they can do to a person's quality of life. Consider that all bodily organs and functions are intricately connected one way or another. In this case, those hormones discussed previously all result from cholesterol. Melatonin is viewed as another important regulator and is needed in the production of these same hormones; UV rays are needed to produce melatonin in the first place. So boom … SUNLIGHT is key!

Look at that: I just solved depression. Ok, not really. However, I want to shine some light on the importance of melatonin production by getting people more exposure to the sun instead of hiding away from it.

Skin cancer!

There I said it, and we all know that it comes from faulty skin cells which, yes, also can be caused by the release of too much melatonin. Remember, the skin is the largest organ in the body with the largest surface area exposed to sunlight and therefore argumentatively is exposed to more free radicals than any other organ (depends on what you eat I guess).

So, there we have it: melatonin is needed to release hormones to prevent depression, fatigue, weight gain, and muscle loss; however, too much can also cause an overabundance of melanin in the skin, which is not good either.

So what am I saying here?

Moderation!

As with anything else in nutrition and health, moderation is your best friend. There is not one thing of which too much is good for you. Even water-soluble vitamin C feeds cancer cells, so too much (even though filtered out through the kidneys and urine) can still have negative effects.

I am simply recommending getting some sunlight, whether from nature or from hitting the tanning bed once a week, to keep your melatonin levels up. Also, sleeping in total darkness helps release melatonin, so shut off that night light.

Funny Thing about Cheating …

Cheat meals are for people out there who work hard all week, eat as healthy as they can, and still like to reward themselves with a cheat meal from time to time.

Some people are pretty strict with their cheat meal and have it the same time every week, no matter what other occasions involving overindulging on processed foods may pop up. For example: people attending weddings may not touch a thing during the reception so that the next morning they can still enjoy their favorite "cheat" cereal.

A while back, I wrote a post about how cheat meals can have a negative effect on the body even though only done occasionally. While I'm not withdrawing that claim, I understand that the society we live in is built on overindulgence. So I am going for the lesser of two evils here, not unlike a needle exchange program for heroin addicts. I am also a firm believer that if you bring a subject to light, people will discuss and gain a better understanding as opposed to ignoring it, feeling ashamed, and doing the wrong thing.

The "cheat" meal isn't used by everybody and I think it's safe to say that MOST people don't incorporate a cheat meal during the week because they live in cheat meal land every day. Every day, the high percentage of the population considered obese or overweight consume food that a health-conscious person wouldn't touch on his worst day. It is not because the food does not smell good, or taste great: it is usually because with knowledge and understanding of the long-term detrimental effects of processed foods, those items are no longer desirable.

No, this blog is about cheating and how a person physically feels once they commit such an act. I currently have a client who wishes she could become so disciplined that she could incorporate a cheat meal. She does not believe she has earned the right to a cheat meal. This thought process is not unique. Along with an overindulgent society we have become a society of guilt. Everything we do that is somewhat pleasurable is deemed as wrong. This occurs to a point where sitting down to actually enjoy a cheeseburger is difficult because of the stigma of eating such food. Many people see eating any "forbidden" food item as enabling a weakness and words like "giving in" and "failure" become a part of their vocabulary of guilt.

I can talk to clients all day about the mental health break a cheat meal can provide to keep the body in a balance of discipline and indulgence. Physical activity breaks throughout the day are recommended. Meditation can reduce blood pressure and lower anxiety. Even just relaxing in nature has many positive impacts on a person's health. So why not choose a pleasurable food item, relax, and enjoy? This vacation from harsh reality can be just what a person needs to stay motivated and positive throughout the week. Incorporating a cheat meal gives a person a workable goal.

The funny thing about cheat meals is that most people are not going to physically feel as good after eating a pizza as they would feel following the salmon salad they usually eat. That physical feeling is also a positive aspect of the cheat meal. Feeling like crap after eating such processed, desired foods is a constant reminder of why a person does not eat these foods on a regular basis. The foods might sound good throughout the week, especially on a stressful Monday when a coworker brings doughnuts in, but you know better than that now don't you? You now have a little secret ... on Sunday afternoon you get to pig out (hopefully guilt-free) on pancakes and bacon because that is what you earned. I like to tell my clients that when you choose to do something, such as eating a cheat meal, it puts you in control. When a coworker brings doughnuts in and you feel overpowered by the immediate pleasure of doughnuts, then giving in is no longer a willing choice, but rather an impulsive decision that is nearly always regretted later.

The thought process is what controls our entire being, so why not strengthen the thought process to including a focus on incorporating healthy foods? Allowing a cheat meal every once in a while allows a person to stay motivated, but also to enjoy the fruits, or "doughnuts" of this life.

Getting out of BED!

Binge Eating Disorder (BED), classified in The Diagnostic and Statistical Manual of Mental Disorders Version 5 (DSM-V), affects more people than any other eating disorder. This manual is the bible that counselors rely on for helping diagnose conditions. Essentially, it works like this: before health insurance will pay for a client's counseling sessions, a diagnosis meeting criteria in the DSM-V needs to be established. This serves as a baseline from which goals can be developed and treatment modalities can be recommended.

The DSM-V 5 defines BAD as:
"a pattern of disordered eating which consists of episodes of uncontrollable eating. During a binge eating episode, a person rapidly consumes large quantities of food. Or a person may consume normal amounts of food so quickly and mindlessly that this would be classified as a binge. Often the binge eating functions help the sufferer manage overwhelming emotions or stressful life events. Binge eaters feel powerless and are unable to control their consumption of large quantities of food. Some people may engage in single episodes of binge eating while others may binge throughout the day."

Symptoms include:

- Uncontrolled consumption of food even when full
- Obsessive thinking or talking about body weight, shape, size, appearance or food
- Depression, anxiety, or extreme mood swings
- Unstable weight
- Eating alone or secretive eating because of embarrassment or guilt
- Rapid eating pace, mindless eating
- Self-criticism, low self-esteem, or feelings of worthlessness

- Urges or desires to consume more and more food
- Body dissatisfaction, body image distortion
- Rituals around body checking, exercise, or food
- Loss of interest in activities, relationships or people
- Large quantities of money spent on food, restaurants, or at the grocery store
- Hoarding of food
- Hidden food or food wrappers

Now, to the treatment of such a disorder. As long as the treatment modality is researched and approved, it is acceptable to apply to the disorder. The theory I choose to utilize with BED is Cognitive Behavioral Therapy or CBT. CBT takes into account thoughts and actions leading to choices that are ultimately classified as BED. When we no longer have evidence of the symptoms, then we are meeting our treatment goals.

The biggest issue surrounding BED is the loss of conscious control when eating. Unfortunately, in a society that seems to encourage over consumption, BED might be more prevalent than anyone would like to admit. In fact, as mentioned earlier, BED is more common than anorexia and bulimia. Many BED symptoms, including eating alone in secret and hiding food wrappers, reveal a deep level of shame. In a previous post I wrote about the "cheat" meal which is essentially a binge (albeit a planned one) related to over-consuming calories and not paying attention to our body's physiological response of being full. This should be conscious and appreciated instead of out of your control.

Discussing a person's existing daily routine, then replacing it with a new daily routine may be one treatment step taken toward combatting BED. For example, if a person's current routine is to eat an apple for breakfast, a bowl of lettuce for lunch, but after getting home from work, consume two enchiladas, chips, crackers, chocolate chip cookies, ice cream, leftovers, and an egg ... now we have pinpointed the typical time at which the pattern runs off course. This person is clearly binge eating and has lost all control. What should be a relaxing, enjoyable experience has consumed them emotionally and mentally as they literally consume food beyond a physical satiation point. While in most cases the food will be highly processed and nutrient deprived it is not necessarily so. Interestingly, the brain is not triggering this hunger response causing the binge, and nutritional knowledge alone won't help it.

As one component of the overall BED treatment plan, nutritional counseling can help. With my own clients, I discuss the importance of regular meals, not only for the various benefits I have discussed in previous blogs, but to maintain blood sugar and gain control of one's appetite. A person who is actually hungry and suffers from a disorder is comparable to adding gas to an already raging fire. Everybody gets burned. By incorporating foods that are beneficial and learning when and why to eat them, we can begin to define and establish healthy eating habits. Additionally, incorporating CBT and an exercise routine further strengthen the efficacy of a total treatment plan.

Exercise releases dopamine, provides activity around which to structure one's day, and helps regulate blood sugar (therefore hunger). Anything that positively impacts a bodily response will further help a person better deal with emotions connected to an embarrassing and possibly debilitating disorder.

Remember: it takes an estimated 3,000 extra calories to put on one pound of body fat. If a person consumes 4,000 calories in an hour (pizza, chips, ice cream, bread, etc.,), and this happens on even a semi-continuous basis then the result will be significant weight issues adding to a person's downward spiral.

If you feel you meet the criteria for this disorder, do not wait another minute. Set up an appointment for counseling assistance. Again, do not feel alone in this and if you are hiding out, putting on excess weight, and feeling that food has control over you, then let me help you "get out of BED" and back to living an enriched life.

Let's Not Get Too Technical …

Separating all fact from fiction that exists about nutrition in this world can be daunting. There seem to be twists and turns at every corner. Eventually you grab the hand of someone who seems to be a helpful friend (or in this analogy, a "diet") then all of a sudden this "friend" leaves you in the dark. You are left alone and without the right knowledge and information needed to get back on track.

Diets, nutrition, food, eating disorders, exercise, nutritionists, personal trainers, organic, raw … aaaaaahhhhhhh!

THERE IS SO MUCH TO LEARN. I CAN'T POSSIBLY BE A HEALTHY PERSON WITH ALL OF THE BS OUT THERE!!!!!!

Some people are constantly bombarded. Every day there is news about a new nutrient or fad fruit or vegetable that needs to be incorporated in your diet if you want to lose weight or gain muscle.

Let me just stop you right there and remind you that food companies make up a multi-billion dollar-a-year empire that controls everything we do. Whether we are talking about lobbyists in Washington, D.C., or bright, colorful food packaging that claims to have everything we need in a convenient box, people need education rather than just relying on companies mass producing foods to tell them what they supposedly need to eat.

Why? Because there is so much more to it than that!

Let's talk about nuts, specifically almonds. When I recommend almonds to clients as a healthy fat source that is all they remember. They don't really care about the extra vitamins, minerals and fiber that this nut provides. As Americans, we have been desensitized to the importance and significance of vitamins and minerals due to all of our advertised processed foods being "fortified" with vitamins and minerals.

The next time you walk down the produce aisle, look for the big colorful ads for tomatoes, kale, or sweet potatoes among other vegetables and fruits. Chances are you will not find any because whole foods do not get to advertise like packaged foods!

Yet walk down the cereal aisle and read all of the boxes and labels that claim their cereal is made with whole wheat, fortified with vitamins and minerals and whatever the newest craze is at the time. Antioxidants, omega-3s, vitamin D, you name it: the cereal companies can refine and add it to their cereals along with another spoonful of sugar for good measure. God forbid anything tastes fishy.

Now, what products are people most likely going to buy? Fortified foods featuring big flashy advertisements and claims, or the more wholly beneficial "what you see is what you get" vegetables, meats, seeds, and nuts without the hype?

Something for people to think about is how easy and convenient it is to buy and prepare whole foods these days. I'm not necessarily saying it has to be organic or free-range. However, if you start by making small changes such as incorporating a real food here or there into your diet, you will eventually start to crave these real foods over the highly-processed, carb-rich products you eat now.

Tying Shoes and Eating Food: Connection?

This morning as I stepped into a pair of *Chuck Taylor Converse* shoes, I also happened to be watching a rap music video at the same time. If you asked me what happened in the video I could describe every detail to you with no problem. However, if you asked me to describe what tying my shoes was like, all I could give you is a generic description of what I did. Maybe I would remember another time where I tied my shoes, but this specific time- no way.

After the video was done, I went to the kitchen and, without any special thought process, opened and ate a can of fish, threw away the can, drank coffee, and brushed my teeth. While I do not specifically remember doing this, I can recall it because it's my routine every morning. It is just a habit!

So what is my point?

Habit-driven behavior is developed when we put ourselves on autopilot to complete tasks we have done thousands of times before. Our mind follows a set script according to different situations. For example, at work you might greet your co-workers, sit down at your desk, and get to work without relying on any decision-making skills or first considering any real goals. When you go to the bathroom you may or may not wash your hands without thinking. When you dine out at a restaurant you put a napkin in your lap without realizing it. You may also wake up, skip breakfast, and then eat a high fat, carb-rich lunch without a second thought.

Yes, the foods we eat may be the result of habit-driven responses from the countless times we have made the same decision in the past. Maybe the smell of a doughnut or the sight of a cookie causes us to grab and consume one while unaware of what just happened. Here's where the script gets more dramatic: when we are chronically overweight and turn to food for comfort when stressed, sad, happy, or angry. Without thinking, we grab something sugary. (I believe this is how the soda industry survives.)

The challenge is replacing this habit-driven behavior with new goals and behaviors. How about goal-driven behavior instead? Goal-driven behavior is where I consciously decide I am going to eat a salad instead of a sandwich; I decide on dressing and extra ingredients: ranch or no ranch, croutons or tomatoes, or both. (I do not recommend the croutons.)

Turn off the autopilot! Make some decisions!

Change whatever you want to change about yourself. Just be aware that habits can be difficult to break, so bring that sledge hammer along whenever you are ready for some real results. Soon enough those goal-directed changes will become habit. Then we're on the right track!

Zonulin ... We Need to be Knowin'!

I have already posted a few times about gluten and the detrimental effects to both the mind and the body that have been exposed in research. I want to be more specific here and put a word out there that people should become more familiar with.

Whether you have a serious disorder, such as Celiac Disease, gluten intolerance, a wheat allergy, Crohns Disease, mind fogginess, difficulty concentrating, or constant diarrhea and stomach aches, then maybe we need to not only identify the products containing gluten in your diet, but learn why this is occurring. After all, knowledge is power!

So the word of the day is: Zonulin!

This little ingredient is what causes the intestinal walls to be opened and exposed to toxins in the bloodstream. It also causes the blood-brain barrier to open up allowing toxins normally filtered through the kidneys and excreted out the body to pour into the brain.

Ouch! Talk about a headache, or maybe something more severe than that! Maybe, just maybe, when you are pregnant and continue to eat wheat sources of carbohydrates the resulting gluten and Zonulin creates a pathway for the same excreted wastes to leak into the baby's umbilical cord and placenta leading to a possibility of birth defects or brain disorders.

In my opinion, pregnancy-related issues surrounding food are analogous to a bricklayer who uses poorly-made bricks that do not hold up very well. While the bricklayer can do his job, much like a mom's body does in growing a baby and giving it all the proper parts, how long is that building going to last as it begins to age? After all, the original materials were cheap and not guaranteed for proper structure or development over the long haul.

Autism has been linked to gluten consumption (along with a lot of other possibilities to be honest) during the developmental growth stages. Yes, bread seems to be everywhere and for some people the thought of not eating a sandwich or crackers with soup is out of the realm of possibility. However, if only for a few months during pregnancy, you could lay off of wheat products to ensure the healthiest baby you could have, then you are doing your job as the best caretaker you can be.

This post is not necessarily about gluten and pregnancy, but more about Zonulin and familiarizing readers with the scientific reason why gluten has the damaging potential it does. Yes, there are some people who eat bread every day and have no (visible) issues whatsoever. However, there is an inflammatory response to gluten because of contaminants, such as Zonulin, that weakens the barrier that separates the digestive tract from the blood stream. You know, that barrier that protects the brain from direct toxins in the bloodstream? Yeah, that barrier. Some people just handle gluten better than others, but there is no amount of working out or dieting that can rid the body of this toxin. The only way to avoid the negative effects of gluten is to steer completely clear of it.

Can you imagine the toxins we create from taking medications or smoking and then, by simply eating bread, we weaken the barrier enough to allow those toxins directly into the brain? That sounds horrible to me, like we would just be destroying the brain much more quickly (Alzheimer's, dementia, rise in mental illness) … just saying.

I Want a Divorce … from My Current Relationship with Food, of Course!

Unfortunately, for the rest of our lives we are stuck in a necessary relationship, one we can never escape. Unlike the crazy ex-boyfriend or former girlfriend you regret and were able to leave behind, you simply cannot get rid of food. You need food to live and even though some may "fast and break" from this relationship, it always comes back!

Much like the relationship you choose to have with your significant other, as long as you both treat each other with respect, love and appreciation, then shared long-term gratification can be achieved. Food can either be a B**** or the love of your life that takes care of you.

Those of you who are in a relationship, think about your significant other. Do you respect him or her? Love him or her? Does she love you back? Would you do anything for her? Would she do anything for you?

Simply put: do you feel your relationship makes you a better person or is it draining the life out of you?

Maybe the sex is good so you stay?

If you don't see the connection I am making here, then you are missing the point. In a healthy relationship there is give and take, sacrifice, and an internal reward for doing so. Your relationship with food can be the same way.

Think about fast food: it is fast, cheap, unhealthy, and extremely pleasurable for a short amount of time, but always leaves you feeling dirty and used. I would never say the same for my significant other. She is kind, caring, and makes me feel better about myself. The same goes for the food choices we all make. There are the poor and gut wrenching decisions, and then there are the good-for-us choices that take a little more investment, but provide a lot more reward.

I know what an unhealthy relationship with another person can lead to, and yet, with experience, knowledge, and a little time, these relationships can either resolve themselves or just go away. With food, however, there is no going away once that choice is made. If I continuously indulge in fast, cheap pleasures I am going to catch a disease. Whether it is heart disease from the constant McDonalds I eat at lunch every day or an unmentionable disease from that woman at the bar who ... Well, you see where this is going: in either case it is extremely unhealthy.

Just as I wouldn't recommend hooking up with the easy girl from the bar due to knowing too much about her, I am too aware of the detrimental effects of poor-quality foods and would not mess with that either! Please understand the significant impact that a relationship with food has on your quality of life. Be patient and wait for the high quality girl who is worth the time and effort: the reward will be so much greater in the long run.

Whey-t a Minute There Protein Powder!

So you have decided to work out and need some additional protein sources to aid in muscle growth? (Remember, protein is the only macronutrient that creates the proper nitrogen balance essential for maintaining and rebuilding muscle tissue among other things.) Well, despite the fact that I recommend as much whole and natural foods as possible, a good protein supplement can really be a big help in adding protein to your diet.

However, it is not as easy as running to Wal-Mart and getting the cheapest protein supplement. You could, but realize that if you go cheap enough sometimes you are not getting anything at all. Instead, I recommend spending a little extra money on better quality groceries.

Some protein powders contain additives, such as artificial sweeteners, and genetically-modified-organisms derived from sick or over produced cows that are used as fillers to make the protein weigh more than it is worth. (You will notice many protein powders brag about weight.)

Plus, the only way to make casein, isolate or hydrolysate is to over process the whey thereby weakening its immune system supporting and muscle building components. Casein protein powder (which many people take at night due to its claim of being slow digesting therefore giving longer protein protection and growth for muscles during longer periods of time) is treated with acid.

Soy is another ingredient that is used to make better protein mixes. Check the ingredient labels on almost all protein powders for "soy lecithin."

What is the problem with soy?

1) Many health experts now consider soy to be an ANTI-nutrient because it prevents the body from absorbing other nutrients.

2) It is thought to be estrogenic meaning it can lead to an increase of female hormones in the body. For guys that is just scary.

Preferably, choose whey protein that is derived from grass-fed cows.

Many cows are injected with Bovine Growth Hormone (BGH) to increase milk production. However, it is also these same cows that often come down with diseases. Chances are that if your protein powder doesn't specifically state it is derived from grass-fed cows, you are likely consuming BGH along with other hormones and antibiotics.

Some of the most popular protein products come from non-grass produced whey protein sourced from China, which is thought to have much lower quality control standards than Europe and the U.S.

It can be tempting for people to buy the cheapest protein in bulk they can find, thinking it is the same quality as other protein powders. However, just like the quality of food matters, the more natural (grass-fed) the more beneficial the protein source is. These cheaper whey powders produced in other countries may contain heavy metals, fillers, and again, soy. (Come on guys.)

Organic, grass-fed protein sources are the way to go if you are going to spend the extra money on supplements in the first place. Yes, it does cost significantly more and initially you will not see huge gains or extreme 8-pack abs poking out. In the long run though, you will be healthier. While experts cannot yet tell you what eating protein treated with antibiotics and hormones can do to a person, I don't really want to sit around and see what could happen.

Personally, I want to avoid taking something that can negate the hard work and efforts I put forth to obtain physical results and overall health benefits, and I advise people likewise.

The Price of Entertainment

This evening my lovely wife, Rach, and I are planning on attending *The Wolverine*, a movie I have anticipated since first seeing the preview a few months ago. I just love the big budget entertainment movies with explosions, killing, and some mutant who is behind it all to justify the violence. According to the commercials, it looks like the bad guys started it.

Two tickets to the movie this evening and possibly a soda for my wife will cost around $25. Not bad considering there are definitely more expensive options, such as eating out that can cost at least $50 (if not more) depending on if somebody (she) wants to get a fancy colored drink, priced around $8 alone, but again, justified.

The funny and nutritionally-relatable thought here is that food seems to be at the center of our entertainment world these days. I mean, really consider the last time you did anything that did not involve food or a beverage. Even at bars where minimal food selections are available, people are still willing to pay lots of money for plenty of calories as a way to gain a pleasurable feeling.

I believe that entertainment is America's biggest export. Slowly but surely, the rest of the world is getting our movies, our food, and also our diseases.

Let's look at our plans with another option:

For the $25 we spent on going out to the movie, I could rent a few movies, order a pizza, get a few sodas, not have to dress up, and still save money. This choice also leaves me more stimulated than going to the movies. Why? Because the taste of food elicits a more direct pleasurable response than any other external stimuli.

Consuming processed food stimulates the brain's opioid receptors, increasing dopamine, much like, oh what's that drug called? Oh yeah... HEROIN. Yes, the pleasurable sugary, starch-rich foods that I like to consume on a cheat meal can provide as much pleasure as an opioid drug and are much cheaper than going to the movies.

Processed food has become so desired that it is now our number one form of entertainment. The movie industry can sit on its millions for a good film, while the food industry can sit on its billions thanks to the pleasure it provides for people every day. Some people do not watch movies, go bowling, miniature golfing, or partake in any other form of active entertainment, but they sure as heck have to eat. When people want to have a fun night in, what is always going to be included besides a game of Twister? I give you food and drink, ladies and gentlemen.

Here's the challenge: try and have a good time without the food and drink. Yes, the cheap, processed, and nutrient-deprived foods that are consumed for entertainment and stimulation do not cost much money wise, especially compared to seeing a movie in a theater, but the cost to your health can leave you penniless. Stimulating foods are pleasurable and encouraged so taking them out of the realm of an every-once-in-a-while food and turning them into a daily staple causes a deficit to our health.

Be aware, people!

Just remember the next time you are enjoying yourself at a party or watching a movie at home, become aware of what you are consuming to make that experience pleasurable. You do not have to reach for the chips or order a pizza to fill a desire that is actually misinterpreted as a need thanks to the habit you have created when you sit down to watch a movie. Instead, try creating a new habit of simply enjoying your movie or other relaxing activity without relying on food or drink aka external stimuli to make it better.

Days off from work can be difficult if I habitually rely on food as my source of entertainment, as compared with just truly enjoying life for what it really is, spending time with my wife, and seeing a good movie. Challenge yourself to gain a better understanding of yourself and what it takes to really enjoy life without automatically including processed, sweetened, and artificially-made foods as part of that equation.

Welcome to the 75th Hunger Post!
(Not Here, But in the Blog Anyway)

Let's go Katniss!!

Yea, I stole that from the *Hunger Games* movie, *Catching Fire*. If you have not had the opportunity to read the books, I strongly recommend them. Essentially, they are about a government that is in control of the people and the sacrifices these people make in each of the twelve districts to continue to be allowed to have food and products from the other districts. Each district has their specialty products needed to sustain life.

Now, anybody who knows me knows that I am in no way a political person and stay out of most of those discussions due to what I ultimately believe in, that God has a plan for us. There is freedom to choose, however for me to get worked up about government policy is a waste of my energies when the needs of the collective people is what is more important. Who cares what the government says if we as a people do not know what we really want?

For example, everybody complains about government policy related to health care, but I have not heard what people really want or expect our government to do to look out for its people. Another policy I hear complaints about (and even I complain a little about) is regulation on animals and crops produced for food.

Here are my issues with the government on food and drug standards:

- They are too general
- They allow too many pesticides and over production
- There need to be more subsidies for farming
- There need to be grants and subsidies that support more organic farms and encourage crop rotation
- There is too much focus on grain and corn production

Because this is a blog and not a research paper, I will get straight to the point. Crop rotation encourages a natural nitrogen balance for fields used for growing plants. Corn, for instance, uses nitrogen while soybeans help replenish nitrogen back into the soil. Because some people do not have the financial means to be able to rotate crops, they saturate the soil with artificial nitrogen sources. These unnatural products leech nutrients from the soil and, used in combination with pesticides, leads to crops that are less resistant to natural pests and weeds. Crop roots may become shallow, getting fewer nutrients found deep in the ground. After generations of this kind of farming, plant/crop sources become nutrient deprived.

People need to step back and appreciate what plants do for the human race. Without the availability of these various crops we simply would not be here. All energy comes from the sun; however, plants are the only organism that can convert this sunlight to carbon that is then used for energy by humans, or animals consumed by humans. Appreciation of and more money spent on this process can only help eradicate some of the chronic diseases that are spreading throughout our society: cancers, autoimmune diseases, blood diseases, and any disease that the body is only able to fight and/or recover from when receiving maximum amounts of nutrients. The more nutrient -deprived foods we are forced to feed people (due in part to governmental control), the more difficult it is to prevent these diseases.

With crops such as corn receiving the most money per yield, farmers don't have the financial freedom to grow anything else. Farmers are also forced to grow the highest yielding crops through whatever available means, including planting hybrid seeds, using pesticides, and adding nutrients: all leading to the depletion of soil's natural nitrogen.

The key to completing this puzzle is to plant different crops and rotate them to restore the nitrogen naturally back into the soil. So, for this 75th hunger post I want people to recognize and respect farmers for the absolutely necessary role they play in the planet's survival. Remember, without plants there is no us. We need the government to focus more on farmers and their vital part in helping sustain the world. Food scientists have found out how to make a profit by turning corn into a sustained product that can be used in almost anything from alcohol to sugar to feed for cows that were never meant to eat it. We also need scientists to refocus from turning crops, such as corn, into sustainable food additives, including alcohol, sugar byproducts, and food that is not good for people or livestock, to more alternative fuel sources or some other product because the damage has already been done to natural foods.

Appreciate those farmers. Renew your appreciation for the foods you consume, and respect yourself enough to eat foods that are whole and natural. Remember where all of your food comes from!

The further from the farm, the less nutrient content it has and more processed it has to be: not good!

Whole Foods, and We Aren't Talking Doughnuts!

Weight loss, cancer prevention and cancer fighting properties, natural energy, disease fighting, immunity booster, muscle growth, fights against depression, fights against anxiety, better sleep, better endurance, better explosiveness, more sex drive, etc. ...

Claims made by products these days are pretty extensive and pretty convincing: just what consumers want to hear. Well, I have an idea. Stop writing large checks for "natural" and "healthy" products, and spend more time in the produce aisle of your whole foods or grocery store.

Somewhere along the way, we as a human race thought we could improve on Earth's natural ability to produce energy needed to sustain life. Remember, the plants we eat trap energy from the sun and through photosynthesis convert sunlight into carbon for energy and the animals we consume eat plants containing nutrients that are converted to energy.

Simple, right?

Again, we are a proud human race and we can do better!

I'm not exactly sure what the first product to contain nonfood substances was but I want to blame margarine. This whole food substitute resulted from scientists hydrogenating monounsaturated fats to mimic saturated fats without using all of the high quality, more expensive animal products. Funny thing is, at the time hydrogenated oils were thought to be healthier. Now we all know better! This discovery by food scientists led to the idea that we can make or alter food into what we want.

So began the birth of packaged and preserved foods with a longer shelf life than was ever intended!

Now here we are in 2013 with packaged "foods" so far removed from their natural plant sources. They sit on shelves for years, contributing to peoples' growing poor health conditions and subsequent illness diagnoses.

It's pretty simple really. Either your body adapts through centuries of changing food sources and modifications, or it becomes sick and weakened trying to do so: survival of the fittest. Essentially, we are at the dawn of the evolution of humans who are either able to synthesize food byproducts or will die trying to adapt to food so devoid of the very nutrients, vitamins and minerals naturally found in whole foods that it might as well be plastic.

So what's next here? Do you want to lose weight, look and feel better? Whatever your wish, the simple answer is to go old school and eat plants and whole food sources. Incorporate whole (meaning one ingredient) foods into your diet and allow your body to receive its necessary nutrients in more absorbable forms.

Diet pills, long stretches of working out, eating disorders, fad diets, starvation, even "diet" foods are all part of the problem, not the recovery. Not a shake that contains so-called nutrients, not a supplement that claims to contain all of the necessary ingredients for the body, not even the food that advertises how healthy it is for you. Guess what? I can beat any packaged shake with Mother Nature's food source straight from the ground. In many cases my product will contain more antioxidants, probiotics, vitamins and minerals in an absorbable form, not to mention cost less!

Yes, it's a highly researched, well-supported claim what whole foods can do. If interested, read the book <u>The China Study</u> about the biggest study ever conducted on the true benefits of whole foods. Mentally note the terminology and different definitions: WHOLE FOODS contain all we need and then some that cannot even yet be isolated or researched, but are shown to contribute to maintaining optimal health compared with nutrients that are found in supplements and food by-products.

Don't Bite the Hand that Feeds You!!

Ok, I'm going to be honest here for a second and sound hippy-ish (not hipster, never hipster): the world is dying and it is our fault.

Whew, ok I said it. Post over …

Nah, instead I would like to elaborate on this offensive, yet truthful statement. The world was established with limited resources and if we continue to destroy these resources, then, well, we are out of time! However, due to modern medicine, people living longer, population growth, and new farming techniques, the world has become over-populated and survival is not without consequences.

There are only a set amount of resources on this earth, such as nitrogen in the soil, oxygen in the air, and useable groundwater. We are not only using it up, but polluting all elements in record time.

Farmers, whether commercial, private, or government subsidized, produce all of the world's food that is then converted into your favorite meal and/or snack. However, what will happen when all of the soil is depleted of nitrogen and no longer able to fertilize the plants being grown? I mean seriously think about it.

What would happen to the earth's population if food production as we know it grinds to a halt?

The world would come to an end.

So, then, why do we continue to tempt fate by abusing the resources that God put on this green planet? I mean science is great! However science is nothing without the nutrition and basic elements needed to make it happen. Organic matter is produced from plants, but basic elements in the ground are also needed for this equation, nitrogen being one.

There is no definite way to predict whether or not this planet will run out of natural resources just like there is no surefire way to determine the exact nutrients needed for the growth and development of an organism. Some things in nature remain a mystery and can outsmart even the most distinguished scientists who attempt to break down and quantify individually used elements. It cannot always be done.

The mysteries of this planet are what keep it alive and when we abuse and overuse those elements needed to sustain life then we will have to pay the consequences, which, yes, means a decrease in population through Mother Nature's plan, not ours.

Starbucks, the New McDonalds

The success that is the Starbucks sales model nearly drives me insane. The company is based on the premise that people will come in, order a sugary beverage with a little coffee in it and pay $4 without ever questioning the expense. Have we simply stopped demanding quality and started paying whatever amount is asked?

I will tell you that the ingredients Starbucks uses are no more superior than any other restaurant or $2 coffee drink found at lesser known coffee shops. Rather, it is the name and the brand that keep people coming back. At home, I can throw together sugar, coffee, cream, and Cool Whip to make most of Starbucks' drinks. Yet people seem to value it more when some 19 year-old barista is combining the exact same ingredients in different variations to make the sugary, pricey drinks.

One of Starbucks' most popular drinks is the Strawberries and Cream Frappuccino with whipped cream. While the description is a pretty good one, using the words "rich" and "creamy" and a "good pick-me-up," I am going to describe how I see it: eighteen teaspoons of sugar and more overall calories than a personal pan pizza. I mean just knowing how many people unthinkingly order and consume this drink provides insight into why obesity is running rampant in America. I have heard of "accidental" calories before, but to consume that many: jeesh.

So, then, how else can we celebrate and reward ourselves? Well, first thing I recommend as a counselor is to find simple, non-harmful, enjoyable activities in which you can partake. Reading a book, taking a walk, conversing with friends, working on your house or apartment, taking up crafts or a hobby: those types of activities can be very satisfying without the negative side effects of stimulating foods. Now if we want the additional stimulation of a food or drink, then we just need to be aware of what we are consuming and limit it to a special treat.

The problem is that there is simply too much justification for rewards on a daily basis. I hate to be the bearer of bad news, but there is no other society as self-indulgent as the U.S.A. Most of the typical Western fast food meals and beverages that people consume daily are considered luxuries elsewhere. Why must we consume a $6, 1,000 calorie "coffee" drink every day? What do we get out of this except an insulin spike, sugar rush, eventual energy crash, and, finally, stored body fat? The rate of over consumption is insane in our society and needs to be changed before Starbucks overtakes McDonald's as the company leading to more cases of diabetes and diabetes-related health ailments. As it stands, we all see that Starbucks is well on its way.

Sorry to offer up Starbucks as the sacrificial lamb because there are a million different coffee stores that do the same exact thing with the same enticing, sugary beverages that contain very little coffee and yet sell like … well, Starbucks!

That Craving for Fast Food ...
Oh, What a Hangover!

College football season got underway yesterday and all over the nation people were drinking to celebrate it. Here in Lincoln, Nebraska, the streets might as well be shut down for all the tailgaters and partying that occurs the night of a Husker game. I should know: I worked the bar scene for four years.

I also know that after all of those drinks are consumed, all the fast food has been eaten, and nothing with useable nutrients has been consumed during the past twenty-four hours, a sick feeling often settles in causing a lack of motivation.

We have all been there, waking up at 10 a.m., feeling like nothing in the world sounds good to eat. Then around 3 or 4 p.m. the blood sugar crashes and the only thing that sounds good is fatty, greasy, processed foods!

Foods such as:

- McDonalds
- Amigos
- Burger King
- Sandwich shops
- Pizza
- Doughnuts
- Chinese food
- Mexican food
- Any and all junk foods, if you catch my drift.

How is it that we allow a night (or entire day) of drinking to so easily obliterate our self-control? Physiologically, we feed our bodies one of the simplest sugars a person can consume, alcohol, for a long period of time. Then because we often follow it by either eating no food, or gorging on processed foods (which only makes the situation worse) our bodies crave more sugar to satisfy that need/desire for more processed carbohydrates.

Alcohol (derived from carbohydrates) hits the blood stream quicker than any food-related carbohydrate, thereby raising blood sugar levels. In turn, insulin is released to filter the sugar as it is processed through the liver. Where people are more likely to experience huge energy crashes, they are much less likely to notice when intoxicated.

An excellent hangover remedy is as simple as warm water with a little honey in it. Why? Honey best mimics the sugars in alcohol, and therefore best regulates the body's cravings for excessive amounts of simple sugars. Think about this the next time you wake up early Monday morning and have to go to work, regretting the past two unproductive days, and all for what? To feel like you are a part of the COLLEGE FOOTBALL scene!!!!

Remember: there is always a cost, whether it is excess body weight, lack of motivation, cravings for unhealthy, high calorie foods, a plunge into depression, or a spike in stress (correlating with the hormone cortisol that spikes with alcohol consumption). These are all things to consider as you face managing, yet again, another hangover and deciding what breakfast foods to eat during the late afternoon!

Just because It's Getting Closer to Fall, Doesn't Mean that the Diet Should!

I am writing this on Labor Day and while summer isn't officially over, the first college football games got underway this past weekend, the weather is a bit cooler today, and the Yankee Candles fall fragrances have been burning in this household for weeks. As I write this, the smell of salted caramel is wafting through the air!

I must admit that I am a fall kind of guy. Summer was great and everything, but let's just move on to the next season in the year and take it down a notch.

One of the many reasons I find fall so interesting is the many foods, coffee drinks, football, and attractive warmer clothes associated with it. I don't know whether or not to write about how, as a child, fall meant cookies, breads, baked items, and homemade meals, or how it meant colorful leaves and the relief of cooler weather.

Ok, the fat kid in me has taken over: food it is!

Not only do I run a nutrition support group and meet with clients for private nutritional counseling sessions, but I constantly research different techniques for helping people establish a healthy relationship with food. Look deeper at how people may relate their feelings to foods. Acknowledge how good a bagel or cinnamon roll is- don't deny it- but also remember what it does to your self-esteem, energy, motivation, and outward appearance.

While the nutritionist in me wants to discuss the importance of restraint this time of year—sticking to vegetables, lean meats, healthy fats, and grains – the fat kid in me wants to eat everything, and the counselor in me wants to understand and have a better relationship with food, involving a little give and take. So this next statement should satisfy all parts:

"Baked goods in the fall remind us of comfort and cooler temperatures encourage us to stay indoors. However, do not be fooled by cooler weather, or give into nostalgia. Stick to your healthier nutritional habits that allow you to continue enjoying how great you look, and put off snacking throughout the week to allow yourself a cheat meal on the day you choose."

Fall is a few months long, just like every season, but it includes a couple of holidays which are typically the worst eating times of the year. I am guilty of overeating during the holidays myself, so let's stay on our toes this autumn and avoid the rich, savory, fluffy, moist breads and other baked products in favor of foods that are more beneficial to our physical and mental health.

I want people to feel good without feeling like they are missing out or having to sacrifice foods in the process. I am asking you to think before you act upon eating sugary, carbohydrate-rich foods. Plan for and then establish a time when you can eat and enjoy food without guilt. Do not let yourself down; don't consume anything and everything when you are most lacking motivation or willpower. Instead, choose to control what you are going to eat and when. Then, after you have finished eating what you want, get back on track, eating the healthful, beneficial foods you more typically eat 95% of the time.

Respect yourself and those around you. Go online and look for healthy alternative recipes for the ones loaded with sugar.

For now, enjoy the weather, football games, and time spent indoors with loved ones.

Looking at the World through Nutritional Goggles AKA Seeing "The Truth"

What happens when you change your perspective?

For example: what happens when you really look at a door that you walk through every single day of work? You open the door and enter without thinking; you leave through that same door, day in and day out. Well, now what about that last day of work right before you are moving on to bigger and better things? Might you look at that door differently? Maybe you spent five years at this company and made a lot of close friends that you will no longer see every day. Maybe you hated your job and could not wait to start anew.

Whatever the case, different situations may trigger different perspectives.

Now let us use that same difference in perspective as it may relate to food that is prepared and served very differently depending on locations, preparation methods and situations. Fry it, bake it, microwave it, put cheese on it, put hot sauce on it, it doesn't really matter what you do to this, "food," as people will understand it to be just that and eat it. For example, when some people see the iconic McDonald's signs, they immediately think "food."

Challenge that thought!

Some people's choice of "food" is the fast variety.

For many people, "food" does not consist of one, but more like twenty ingredients. On the contrary, "food" coming from fast food eateries or even sit-down restaurants more often meets the definition of entertainment and stimulation than it would be considered a traditional food.

Where are the nutrients?

Where are the antioxidants, vitamins and minerals?

Where is the color that is supposed to be in all organic materials?

What have food scientists done to this one time plant product?

In place of food, we now have food by-products. Food by-products are killing millions whereas actual food is keeping people alive. Food by-products are responsible for diseases and a growing population of depressed people, while food helps cure diseases and triggers the brain's pleasure-sensing neurotransmitters.

As the blog says, something to think about: this time try to identify and increase the amount of foods you eat and reduce the food by-products. You'll be well on your way to a more satisfying lifestyle.

Sugar, Spice, and Everything … Healthy?

If little girls are made of sugar and spice, where does that leave little boys? How about protein and a moderate amount of unprocessed fats? (I feel like I should make a Spice Girls joke here!) It is a stretch because we all know that girls are not always that sweet, plus by now we know that what is sweet for us is not always beneficial for us.

When I hear the word spice I turn to thoughts, smells, flavors, and recipes that include pumpkin, wafting scents of bakery items and the ever-popular Starbucks PSL (pumpkin spice latte for you non-coffee drinkers out there).

Ok, stick with me here, but spices include various kinds of pepper, capsaicin, thyme, basil, chili, Cajun rubs, turmeric, cayenne, cinnamon, cumin, nutmeg, ginger, curry, fenugreek and many more that can really kick up the flavor in a lot of bland and seemingly tasteless food.

I personally favor cayenne and pepper in my food and, as anyone who knows me can tell you, I put it on almost everything. I know that egg whites mixed with spinach alone just doesn't have very much taste. However, when I add my hot sauce (mostly cayenne and vinegar), I feel I am getting actual taste satisfaction with my meal. My wife hates the smell by the way!

Remember the benefits of colors as noted in previous posts!

When I make a bowl of steel cut oats, I add cinnamon, which enhances the flavor and, as a side effect, helps regulate blood sugar.

Take any shrimp and combine it with Cajun seasonings (minus the sugar), and you have got yourself a tasty Cajun dish. Add a little Quinoa on the side to further compliment the meal. Chili powder is another tasty spice that can complement lean meats, eggs, and fish. Add a little salt and possibly a sweet potato and boom! You have got yourself another healthy and tasty meal.

There are thousands of different combinations of spices to be used with lean meats, complex carbohydrates, and healthy fats that result in healthy and enjoyable dishes.

So, not only can a lot of these spices be beneficial for your salivary glands but your overall health as well. As stated earlier, cinnamon helps regulate blood sugar. Capsaicin (found in chili, pepper, and cayenne seasonings) is great for stimulating the metabolism and is actually a main ingredient in many expensive diet supplements.

Ginger is great for free-radical prevention, heartburn relief, and stopping the growth of cancer cells.

Various spices also have been linked with anti-inflammatory properties which are great detoxifiers when coming off of a typical western diet. Chronic pain, headaches, and bodily aches can be treated by an herbal doctor usually through the use of spices both externally and internally. Just think: many home remedies used by ancient civilizations are artificially produced using the same spices and commercialized, now costing a fortune ... thanks again food scientists! (sarcasm)

So, the next time you complain about a boring dish of "healthy" food, just remind yourself that you must be the boring one. Thanks to a wide range of spices, there are tons of healthy and tasty combinations that also provide nutritional benefits. If you do not believe me, just check Pinterest. (However, avoid the baked goods section).

Brain Food!

While this might not be one of my more popular posts, it is essential information for people wanting to build healthy brains and avoid brain ailments and nerve damage later in life.

Here is a three-step process about how the body breaks down …

1. People consume processed foods, smoke, avoid exercise, spend little to no time doing stimulating mental exercises, and expose themselves daily to toxic chemicals and environmental conditions … all leading to free radical damage and oxidation in the brain and throughout the nervous system.
2. Further compounding the free radical damage and oxidation is the fact that people do not consume enough actual preventative nutrients and antioxidants.
3. Eventually this all leads to degenerative brain diseases, including Multiple Sclerosis, Alzheimer's, and other brain-related diseases that could have been prevented through healthier eating habits and lifestyles.

BUT it is never too late … today is your day to start!

*Omega-3s consist of two long chain fatty acids, DHA and EPA, that are found in fish, grass-fed beef, and chia seeds, for starters, and essentially make up 60% of the brain's ability to function.

So, from the get-go, incorporate more Omega-3s, B vitamins, and antioxidants into your diet. I could get more specific here and also recommend more calcium, iron, folic acid, or specific B vitamins. However, when foods incorporate the "Big 3" they are usually already rich in an array of useful vitamins and minerals, all of which are essential to facilitate brain health. For example, B12 along with folic acid facilitates brain function and manufactures much-needed neurotransmitters. Also, B6 is needed to produce all amino acids (from complete protein sources) that fire up neurotransmitters.*

So this should be easy then!

When consuming fish, fresh spinach, and a bowl of steel cut oats for breakfast, I know that I have not only protected my brain and filled my belly with slow digesting food, but lowered my caloric intake and eaten highly-efficient foods, meaning foods that maximize my overall health, particularly brain health.

All brain cells (neurons) are developed in the womb, meaning there are no more once maturation in the womb is complete. Therefore, all we can do with what we have is to form proper neural pathways, which can be strongly impacted by the food we choose to consume. To believe that after we are born we can eat whatever we want, do drugs, negate sleep, and spend limited time on learning and neural stimulation but still form a peak performing brain is not accurate.

Many mental disorders result from environmental factors that cause genes to behave (or express) improperly. For example, what if an expectant mother had followed a regimen of getting all of the essential nutrients in balance while abstaining from smoking, drinking, and drugs, and getting plenty of sleep? Then it is possible and more likely that her fetus would develop a brain free of mental illnesses.

Once a baby is born with its delicate bundle of neurons (the brain), that organ is shaped by its environment and the decisions of its caretakers. Environment in this instance includes the amount of affection and physical touch the baby receives, as well as proper nutrition and safety. No matter how much money a family has, or how expensive the house in which they live or car that they drive, the environment and level of care provided accounts for much more than any external factors than society may equate with a values system. For example, spend more time with the child and less time making money. Spend more money on quality food, and less on "things" or "stuff" to elevate us in the eyes of friends and neighbors.

Remember, the period in which a fetus' brain is developing requires proper nutrients from whole foods as well as a safe, calm, stress-free environment to develop. The same things could be said for babies, children, youth and adults: instead of relying on SSRIs, mood stabilizers, anti-psychotics, sleep aids, anxiety and depression medications, we need to prescribe diets early on to prevent illness and brain oxidation, and to establish healthy neural pathways that account for positive, calm, and focused brains that release proper amounts of neurotransmitters.

All of these factors can start with wild fish, dark green leafy vegetables, and a bowl of steel cut oats for breakfast. Maybe this could be your new medicine. If you are anything like me, maybe you will start to enjoy and figure out new, inventive ways to doctor up your medicine to make it more enjoyable (like hot sauce).

*Quick reminder here: neurotransmitters are what make people feel, think, and act the way they do. The big three are serotonin (which provides calm, long-term satisfaction, attention), dopamine (which provides pleasure), and norepinephrine (excited, anxious). There are others, such as acetylcholine, which is used to contract muscle fibers; however, this post is more about behavior and thought process due to the brain's health.

Marathon Eating ... Revisited

Today, my wife and I had the pleasure of running 13.1 miles in the Omaha Half Marathon. I must say I was a bit disappointed by a few things: the turnout compared to the one here in Lincoln, Nebraska; the MC who was yelling at 7a.m. for everyone to "get back;" the loop at the end of the race through a baseball field that came out of nowhere; and finally the lack of a big ol' pizza or some other unhealthy yet stimulating reward post-race, which didn't happen.

Yesterday in preparation for this long run, I consumed massive amounts of ca ... nah not carbs, but dark green leafy vegetables full of vitamins, minerals, and antioxidants that lowered my acidity, allowing me to retain less water and maintain a balance of fluid throughout my run today. Usually, it is believed that a run like this (especially for someone my size) will burn such a large amount of calories that extra carbohydrates are needed. I disagree, and I think other serious runners should too.

I can't help but touch on the myth here that "carb-ing up" the night before a race is essential to a successful run. In actuality, all that leads to is storing extra fat due to the amount and simplicity of the carbohydrates typically consumed the night before a race, like pasta, rice, or a form of bread. Simply put, those carbohydrates consumed the night before will not stay as converted muscle glycogen until the morning, forcing the leftover glycogen to reprocesses through the liver and convert to body fat.

While the idea of "carb loading" exists, it means that your body must first be carbohydrate deficient or in fasting, which in turn affects your recovery and training energy leading up to the race. To properly "carb load" one must taper down the carbohydrates and continue with the same intensity of workouts until almost all muscle glycogen is completely drained out of the system. This then allows the body to utilize fewer carbohydrates and store large amounts more long-term (a few hours).

This is supposed to shock the body when people finally consume pasta, bread, or rice (again the usual carbohydrate-rich foods for runners). However, if not doing this correctly, you have just consumed a large amount of processed carbohydrates for no reason resulting in water retention, discomfort and bloat. You'll be one of the people standing outside the port-a-potties on mile 6.

Remember, fatty pasta meal is really equivalent to dairy+fat+simple carbohydrates the night before, and result in visits to the port-a-potty on race day.

Runner's nutrition does not have to consist of simple carbohydrate sources with hardly any vitamins, minerals, or long-term benefits for recovery and sustainability for the next activity. I consumed a regular amount of steel cut oats the night before with egg whites and spinach then went to bed while sipping on water. As a result, I did not feel uncomfortable while sleeping or upon waking.

Consume a regular portion of a complex carbohydrate source with minimal fiber and add some coconut oil to extend the life of your breakfast.

Remember, you participate in running events to be healthy and have a good time. Don't turn it into an excuse to over consume, or possibly worse, get diarrhea. There are many variables that cause people to perform well. Training properly and eating to train and recover properly will establish an efficient body that will accomplish a race without excess energy just waiting to be stored.

So, for the next run try veggies, healthy fats, and lean protein sources the day before the run. I would recommend eating many small meals throughout the day. I do not recommend eating a large pre-run evening meal, which will only spike insulin levels and leave a person feeling more lethargic than normal. The morning of the race, consume less fibrous carbohydrates along with a good protein source and maybe some healthy fats, such as rice with egg whites or a moderate protein supplement and a few fish oil capsules, or my favorite, coconut oil in my rice. This will help feed muscles and sustain blood sugar levels throughout the race. Consuming carbohydrates alone could cause a blood sugar crash before you are even out of the gate. I would consume a little caffeine for a burst of energy for those early races as well as endurance (which research as shown for it to be effective). Lastly, I would consume more fluids the week leading up to the race.

Saturday, September 28, 2013
Birthday (remixed)

September 28th, just another day … however, I was born on this day 28 years ago. Thanks mom and dad!

On this day 28 years ago, the world was changed as it is changed and altered with every single person born. I would like to believe the world is a little better with my birth and life, but who really knows?

So, what am I going to do to celebrate my birthday?

Probably eat some fish, vegetables, and drink some … water. MMM … my kinda birthday!

Yes, as deprived as it sounds, I try not to see it that way. I cannot help but question why society started to incorporate food as a celebratory fixture for a holiday that celebrates life. I know from the minimal research I have done on birthday cakes that this tradition of incorporating a "cake" dates back to Ancient Roman times. However, they did not have the ingredients we have because certain foods had not yet been "invented" (yes, we "invent" foods now). Modern birthdays have become an excuse for gluttony and overconsumption, especially in our Western culture. Just think about birthday parties as a kid: were they not chock full of goodies and sugary drinks? Were birthday cake and ice cream not staples of growing up? Even when you go to a restaurant and your friends think it is funny to tell the waitress it is your birthday just to embarrass you, they bring a complimentary cake out to the table and sing.

Do cultures outside of our own perform this sort of ritual?

I am curious as to why I am considered the deprived one because I choose not to eat birthday cake and ice cream. I enjoy fish and vegetables which are nutritionally satisfying, so there is no problem on my end. However, people close to me think that eating nutrient-rich foods is such a sacrifice. If anything, missing out on sweets and processed foods allows me to enjoy more satisfying parts of life over the long-term, or, from a more scientific point of view, I enjoy serotonin rather than an immediate "dopamine dump" resulting from eating processed foods.

I will be honest: I can see how what I am doing may look as if I am sacrificing my golden birthday (28 on the 28th), but I see it differently and challenge others to do the same. I want people to experiment the next time they are at a social event or celebration: focus on the people you are with rather than the food or drink you are consuming. Really try to understand what it is in life that you enjoy and go for it. I know it may be easier at the time to give in and eat a piece of cake with a big ol' bowl of ice cream because society allows you to justify it. However, why put yourself in a sugar-coma and discount all appreciation of the events going on around you?

At one point I used to look forward to Saturdays, holidays, and celebrations because of the abundance and availability of processed, immediately gratifying foods. Hopefully now I will enjoy other indulgences and pay closer attention to real life.

As for now, let me blow out the candles on my tuna fish and consume a bowl of quinoa after a 5-mile jog and enjoy my birthday. (Who knows, maybe this could be part of a new tradition?)

Feeling Anxious?

If you're anything like me then from time to time you get excited. I mean nervous. I mean anxious. I mean worried. Wait...

Maybe you're sitting at your coffee table right now and you're twitching your foot as you drink your fourth cup of coffee in an hour and wondering why you have four tabs open on your computer, music in the back ground, and are attempting to get three things done at once.

Maybe not ...

Maybe you're getting that butterfly feeling in your stomach much like right before you asked that pretty girl in high school to prom but yet you're just trying to read a book.

Either way, if you know what I'm talking about, then you might be struggling with anxiety.

Anxiety is defined as:

"stress that can come from any event or thought that makes you feel frustrated, angry, or nervous. Anxiety is a feeling of fear, unease, and worry. The source of these symptoms is not always known."

Again, I am not talking about the excitement and anticipation for something good, but the worry that something bad will happen when there is no rational reason to believe so. In most cases, if something "bad" did happen it is actually easier to deal with than the worry of it possibly happening.

For those of you who struggle with anxiety much like I have my entire life let me recommend some natural things for you to try to reduce anxiety:

- Chamomile (tea)
- L-theanine (found in green tea)
- Hops (yes the kind found in beer)
- Valerian Root (this stuff is also used as a sleep aid)
- Lemon Balm

- Passionflower (remember a passion fruit flavored drink is not the same)
- Lavender Oil (smell it)
- Omega-3s (yes the fishy kind of oil)

Along with these natural nutrients that can be found in food, there is always the option to hold your breath, sweat, exercise, remain mindful of your surroundings, and of course, breathe deeply.

I recommend taking these natural remedies into consideration prior to losing too much sleep, getting too worked up, or negatively impacting your own quality of life by catastrophizing everything. The truth is (and you know this in your rational state of mind) getting worked up or anxious has NEVER helped you in the past and it is a complete waste of energy. Yet you have trained your brain to worry and that is its "go to" in times of stress.

Another thing about anxiety, stress, and worry is that it literally stops your metabolism.

Think about fight or flight reflexes which were meant to put our bodies in a readiness state of either freezing to avoid being seen by predators or to fight or run in defense. What does the body need to perform these actions?

Energy!

How much?

As much as it can get.

So, when you start to worry about that assignment due or have that anxious feeling for no particular reason, your body will release cortisol that literally stops the metabolic functioning in your body and sends all resources to the muscles to ready them for an immediate reaction. Stress is no longer a beast or prey in the wild like our ancestors had to deal with and is now a complete waste of energy and stoppage of metabolism. Stress also depletes muscle, causes ulcers, increases body fat, and affects areas of the brain.

So, despite the fact that it is easier said than done ("don't worry about it, what will happen will happen, and oh wells" seem to exist for others),it is up to you to determine if you are going to challenge this anxiety or live in it. If you do begin to worry, get up, get moving, and try some "at home" remedies that can assist you in your journey through life.

Addiction Is Next to Survival

In the counseling world, many people follow the principals of Maslow's Hierarchy of Needs.

The way this little pyramid works is that the higher up the pyramid a person wants to be, they need to first achieve the preceding levels. For example: I am not going to be able to worry about love if I do not have enough food. I need food, water, sleep, and oxygen to survive. (Yes, Maslow does put sex on the NEEDS part of life.)

As counselors, we apply this concept to treatment. When someone is in danger or possibly endangering somebody else, then we must take the appropriate action and report him or her to people who can help. That precedes self-actualization which would be a counseling session.

Another aspect of life that can override damn near anything is addiction.

When your brain becomes addicted to something, it is due to the fact the body now begins to rely on what that "something" can do for that person. For instance, if every day I wake up and drink a 1.75 of vodka, then my brain will begin to adjust in preparation for the alcohol that it expects to consume.

The brain wants to stay in a state of homeostasis which is again on the most basic level of human needs. So, when I stop drinking the bottle of alcohol every day, I get sick and feel the typical symptoms of withdrawal.

The body doesn't like imbalance or extreme change. To help the body from feeling these sometimes devastating feelings the body craves more to prevent imbalance which gets interpreted as pain or discomfort. Some people are able to stop, however some are not. The people who need to continuously feed that craving and build up a tolerance to the point where everyday life is negatively affected are simply called addicts.

Being an addict means that in Maslow's Hierarchy of Needs there is a new priority and it involves eating, sleeping, breathing, and addictive substance. (Yes, it overrides everything.)

Now, think about people in the same light as alcoholics. They are addicted to another kind of sugar. The sweet tooth, the can't-eat-just-one people, the people whose whole desire is to lose weight yet they continuously find themselves at the bottom of a cookie box wondering what the hell happened.

Just remember that you can have a sugar addiction and it can be very detrimental, to the point that you find your quality of life has severely decreased due to the need to fill that sugar craving.

Yes, the craving and desire to fill that void in your life is very real and needs to be treated as such. Do not minimize this if you are a person who desires to kick that sugar to the curb and cannot. This is very real and should be discussed if you feel the need is getting out of control.

One recommendation I have is to put the magazines that discuss weight loss down. You know what your problem is: it isn't meal planning, and it isn't eating your vegetables. It is a constant need for sugar no matter what else is consumed. Do not think to yourself that you can have just a little or maybe a taste.

No my friend, you are an addict and the worst kind too. Your drug is cheap, easy, and, unlike methamphetamine, society loves to push sugar like it's a new diamond ring!

So, if you think you may have that deeper desire for a substance, then you may be addicted. I recommend looking into some appropriate ways to treat this addiction. Research shows that a nutritionist alone may not be able to satisfy what you need for the big picture. The connection between sweets and satisfaction is too strong to be talking proper nutrients and supplementation. No, you need the big guns my friend, you need a Nutritional Counselor!

Damn It Society, You're Killing Me!

So, I think by now that most people understand that you have to be a thin girl or a muscular guy and be extremely attractive to get what you want in this society.

I mean that is what we're meant to believe anyway, according to:

Magazine covers
Social Media
Advertising
Fashion
TV shows
Movies
Even the gym!

It seems as though everywhere you turn all of the successful people, or ones you notice anyway, are the attractive ones with abs and toned arms.

So what happens if you feel you were dealt a sh***y hand and weren't blessed with the looks or body type to get the perceived successful future you covet? My recommendation is to take matters into your own hands, have a good personality, take care of your body to the best of your ability, and enjoy life to the fullest. Forget about some ridiculous standard that nobody can live up to. (After all, we are all familiar with Photoshop.)

So what happens if we aren't strong enough or don't have enough willpower to achieve what we desire so badly? I'm talking about the beautiful, rich, and powerful people.

Some people turn to drugs to assist them with their weight loss and boost their energy levels to accomplish tasks a normal human being could never accomplish by himself.

Drugs are quite popular with society, especially youth for simple things such as losing a little weight, studying longer and harder, and being able to stay awake for days in an attempt to accomplish their perceived goals.

Yes, these highly addictive substances are being abused by young people to assist them in meeting unrealistic standards of beauty and success.

Eventually, using a drug to assist you in doing something extreme to your body leads your brain to compensate for this foreign chemical. This means that your brain expects the chemical and, without it, it begins to "crave" this substance and compensates with withdrawal feelings until the substance is taken again. When this occurs, we are no longer taking a substance to succeed. We are taking a substance to fulfill a need or an addiction. Years go by and you could potentially find yourself in a drug rehabilitation center attempting to piece your life back together, analyzing the series of impulsive choices that led to being homeless with a drug induced psychosis. (Sorry, my mom was a worst-case-scenario type. It's a learned trait.)

Another thing about utilizing substances at a young age is the fact that it stunts the maturity of your brain. So let's say at twelve years old you began using meth on a regular basis until your twenties. Once you do stop, your mature age will be stunted at the age you started using the substance. So now not only are you troubled with addiction, but your brain and emotions aren't where they should be, leaving you with social concerns.

Although this scenario doesn't happen to everyone and as a matter of fact most people will not fall into addiction, it does happen. Remember, there is no gene that is yet identified to target in treatment of addiction that can be "fixed." So, if society is pressuring you to be thin and you do "whatever it takes" to get there, just remember that there is always a cost for any severe and harsh changes the body goes through.

Yes, I know people personally who started using methamphetamine, cocaine, and especially Adderall to assist them in their weight loss and career goals. Now they are burned out, miserable, in poor life situations, and have put themselves in unfortunate situations that they will never forget.

The pressure to take the "easy route" will always be there, as well as the pressure to "push yourself." Balance is key, and long-term consistency in eating and working out can assist in your life goals. For the here and now, put the Cosmo magazine down, quit beating yourself up, and talk to someone. Talk to a counselor, friend, family, someone.

Do not isolate!

Benefits of Eating

Benefits of eating… right?
Benefits of eating … raw?
Benefits of eating … Paleo?
Which is it?

Well, truth be told, the benefits to eating start right there with eating. Our primal, hunting and gathering ancestors had issues with food, but it was more so with just getting enough. So, every day the sole purpose was to obtain food so that the people of that tribe could continue to live.

Fast forward a couple of years and now the human race has developed food that can sit on store shelves for years and years… and years. The norm is to have food ready in 2 minutes as opposed to foraging all day to survive. The standards have dropped for survival and the Western Diet has become reliant on technological advances to provide for our needs.

This isn't a bad thing; however it is just natural evolution of a developing people. In all fairness, it is good for us that we have cured hunger and malnutrition – or have we?

Food is consumed for the basic reason to give the body essential nutrients to survive. Nutrients are "essential" because the body cannot produce all that is needed to sustain life. The body needs nutrients from an external source (food) to form metabolic reactions, for the brain to function, repair, and maintain homeostasis.

So, you can imagine what would happen if someone went through life with inconsistent and sporadic eating?

I mean yes, one general idea is that calories spread evenly throughout the day can provide the body with constant nutrients that allow the body to maintain. However, if you are a person (much like my wife) where your day completely engages your interests and you become so busy that eating is an afterthought, then it is very hard for the body to compensate for these drastic changes and malnutrition can occur.

Another example of malnutrition is when people struggle with substance abuse. If you have the opportunity to sit down and talk with a meth addict for example, you will begin to develop an idea of the horrors they have done to their body and how it's a wonder that the body even functions. One of the biggest concerns with meth use is that you can go days without sleeping or eating which are two essentials to sustain life. I can't even begin to fathom all of the damage that can be caused by lack of eating alone, not to mention lack of sleep, ingesting a toxic substance, and exposure to various diseases.

Yes, meth use is an extreme example, but what should be encouraging to most is how resilient the body can be. Like I said, it is amazing that, with treatment of course, an alcoholic or drug addict is still capable of performing basic life skills, not to mention still able to achieve difficult goals. So though the body prefers homeostasis, it can bounce back from some pretty major issues. However, going too long in a malnourished state makes the body's ability to recover lessen over time.

If you are one of those, "inconsistent" people who go through life constantly abusing the body by barely eating, substance abuse, lack of sleep, or elevated stress, then you may be having some of the largest health detriments any over-eater/overweight person will ever experience. Not eating will literally destroy your body quicker than anything else. The body is constantly rebuilding and needs nutrients to do so. Without these essential nutrients, the body simply cannot do what it needs and health ailments are quick to follow.

So, if you are starting out on a "diet" or some other way of trying to live healthier, remember the first rule to any nutrition plan:

Eat!

The rest can be filled in later!

Willpower, the Last Line of Defense!

Are you one of those people who struggle to understand the guy who gets up at 5 AM in the morning, eats a nutritious breakfast, and then heads to the gym?

Do you look at him and desire that type of willpower in your own life?

Or maybe you ARE the guy who gets up for the gym but sees that girl who pays all of her bills as soon as she gets them?

Either way, we can always look up to another person, see what they are doing, and desire the will to do that thing.

At its essence, willpower is the ability to resist short-term temptations in order to meet long-term goals. And there are good reasons to do so. University of Pennsylvania psychologists Angela Duckworth, PhD, and Martin Seligman, PhD, explored self-control in eighth-graders over the course of the school year. The researchers first gauged the students' self-discipline (their term for self-control) by having teachers, parents and the students themselves complete questionnaires. They also gave students a task in which they had the option of receiving $1 immediately or waiting a week to receive $2. They found students who ranked high on self-discipline had better grades, better school attendance, higher standardized-test scores, and were more likely to be admitted to a competitive high school program. Self-discipline, the researchers found, was more important than IQ in predicting academic success.

I struggle when I see people who have the willpower to keep everything clean and organized when I let it slip by in busy times.

So what is it exactly about WILLPOWER that makes it so useful in determining success in things we desire to do?

Lack of willpower can lead to us continuing old habits, in fact …

Lack of willpower isn't the only reason you might fail to reach your goals. Willpower researcher Roy Baumeister, PhD, a psychologist at Florida State University, describes three necessary components for achieving objectives:

First, he says, you need to establish the motivation for change and set a clear goal.

Second, you need to monitor your behavior toward that goal.

The third component is willpower. Whether your goal is to lose weight, kick a smoking habit, study more, or spend less time on Facebook, willpower is a critical step to achieving that outcome.

So, currently my motivation is to lean up for a bodybuilding show. My clear goal is to achieve 3% body fat.

My behaviors toward this goal consist of eating right, working out, restricting alcohol, sugar, and processed foods, as well as doing my research to better understand how my body utilizes carbohydrates vs fats vs proteins as opposed to what I need to get my body fat to an elite level.

There are various other things I need to do achieve these small objectives. I need to go grocery shopping at least once a week, prepare my meals, wash my gym clothes for the morning, take recommended supplements, eat my vegetables, monitor my energy levels to make sure I am not just burning calories but burning mostly fat instead.

Now, I need the willpower to complete the above steps.

Everybody knows that setting a goal and completing one are two completely different things. I recommend that when you set a goal, don't set it and forget it, but make a plan like I just did where I addressed the steps I need to take to help achieve that goal. No goal is unrealistic; however, some may be more long-term and take more investment. I recommend long-term goals but understand that small goals need to be achieved to keep a person motivated.

An example of setting short-term goals to help achieve long-term accomplishments is when people eat healthy. The goal is that from day to day, people that eat healthy feel better than those that don't. So, the short-term goal achieved here is to just feel better every day. This then helps meet the long-term goals of weight loss and practicing better eating habits.

Simply put: if what you are doing is not working towards that goal, then it's wrong. For instance if I talk about lowering my body fat, but then you catch me at Pizza Hut, then clearly I lost the willpower at that moment to achieve my goals.

Think about the commercials or advertisements in magazines of the people getting up early, working out, and looking good and confident throughout the day. These always look enticing until YOU are the one who has to get up and get going.

This is where your willpower comes into play.

Honestly, if you have all of the short-term steps prepared such as a meal, clothes laid out, gas in the car, gym bill paid etc., then you are making that choice (or exercising your willpower) to accomplish your goals a little easier.

After some time of using sheer willpower to wake up in the morning to lift, run, get to work on time, get to yoga, kick boxing class, or whatever else your goals consist of, you will eventually establish a habit, one that will become second nature. This is truly how "those people" you see get up in the morning and keep working so hard are able to keep doing it. It's second nature. Now, when it comes to pushing past your usual limits such as getting your body fat dangerously low like I am attempting, then willpower will be what drives me: the will to be the best, the will to win.

You can see over time that willpower turns into a habit!

Next thing you know, goal achieved, and you can establish another one.

How to Make "Healthy" Food Taste Good

This is a build off of a recent post. I took information from a book written by Dr. Kessler, <u>The End of Overeating: Taking Control of the Insatiable American Appetite,</u> to describe what the food industry actually does to food material to not only stimulate our various senses, but to actually override the system with pleasure. The combinations the food scientists come up with are what keep people coming back for more, even when not experiencing true hunger.

This concept of experimenting with food doesn't have to be done in a lab. It can be attempted in our own kitchen with a few basic principles.

This is where things are pretty simple.

The concepts from Dr. Kessler's book are that there are three to four main ingredients (if counting alcohol) that make food so stimulating.

These are: fats, sugars, salts, and alcohol.

Keep those 4 things in mind because that same principal applies when trying to make food more palatable.

Let's take an example of a meal of chicken breast and broccoli. Now, by themselves they can be pretty boring. They are boring because there are minimal fats, no additional salt, and not enough sugar in these food items (minus the minimal natural sugar in the broccoli of course). So, do I continue to eat this dry and unsatisfying food for months so that I can walk around the poolside for a few days this summer?

No silly, we need to make this food palatable by following our rules of nutrition:

1. Attempt sauces that are sodium based. No added sugars and certain plant oils are approved.

2. Added sweeteners is not preferred; however, they can make a large amount of difference in taste without adding calories.
3. Fats add texture and satisfaction that can be just enough to get through a dry meal.
4. Drink plenty of water. (Always true.)
5. Attempt to cook food in various ways (bake, boil, microwave, etc.). This can change the texture/taste just enough to make a difference.
6. When in doubt, add a little fat to the diet. This naturally adds texture and a little natural sweetness as well.
7. When there is something fat (cream, nuts, seeds, coconut oils, etc.) add just a little sweetness and the combination can make for a great dessert.

Ok, I just made these rules up, but by following them you will notice they can really help out.

Take rule number five for example. I have a client that was eating raw almonds and drinking a protein shake in the evening. I asked if he had ever reduced the almond milk in the shake, then added the almonds and blended them together. Then take that mixture which is thick with fats, minimal liquid, and sweetened from the protein powder and put it in the freezer for a few hours. Next thing you know, you have an ice cream-like dessert that stays completely within the confines of what you were eating anyways.

Take number seven now and apply that principal to a dessert. Maybe take an unflavored Greek yogurt (protein and bland), mix with some stevia, and then add a tablespoon of peanut butter. If you want to get crazy, add a little cocoa powder (unsweetened of course).

Bam!

Now you have a thick pudding consistency that is full of protein, healthy fats, and can be eaten at any time of the day.

Number one is a principal I apply every day of my life because I utilize hot sauce on almost all of my food, including oatmeal. In this rule, people question sodium content and to this I state that once you remove all processed and packaged foods from the diet, sodium levels drop significantly. Drink plenty of water (rule four) and eat green veggies high in potassium and you will not have any issues with the added salt from a hot sauce or salsa. In fact, there is no documented research that shows adding table salt to foods is linked to elevated blood pressure.

Rule number six is one that can add a little more calories but can significantly increase satisfaction in your life. I use this example with fish. Many people do not like fish simply because it tastes "fishy" and there are minimal fats in most fish. So I recommend when baking fish to use some real mayonnaise and then sprinkle some parmesan cheese on top. Next, allow that to bake and form a crust which can add texture and flavor. Bam again! Happiness.

Other rules such as adding a fat source to a fiber source (apples and peanut butter), high fiber alternatives (chia seeds and flax seeds to add bulk), and a few berries for added sweetness in a bland anything really, yes even lean meats (try some blueberries mixed in your lean meats patties next time).

These simple rules will help you understand that just because the guy in the magazine is pictured eating a dry chicken breast and dry brown rice, doesn't mean that you're stuck with that to live healthy.

For healthier recipe alternatives you can follow me on Pinterest under my board "recipie for success" (yes I spelled it wrong on purpose)

Forget Bananas, Let's Go Coconuts!

At this point in the news most people have at least heard or possibly caught on to the coconut craze. I mean you see coconut in everything now: coconut milk, shredded coconut in recipes, coconut extract for healing purposes, coconut flour, coconut sugar, coconut vinegar, coconut water... so much so that I sound like "Bubba" talking about shrimp.

There is a reason that coconuts have become so popular and for the purpose of this post, it's mainly the oils. This is due to the fact that coconut oil is part of a class of oils called MCTs or medium chain triglycerides. If you are immersed in the athletic world, then you have heard of or possibly bought MCT oil for its "fat burning" properties. I know that now as I see more and more coconut oils on the shelves of even Wal-Mart, people are now getting a healthy dose of MCT, which means we should all be getting thinner right?

Again, not that easy.

According to Dr. Laurie Cullen at the Women's Institute, when MCT's are absorbed into the blood stream they bypass the digestion process that longer chain fats go through (such as the Omega-3s I love so much). MCTs are said to provide quick energy for the body and are less likely to be stored as fat. Also the thermogenic effect of food when consumed with MCTs is said to increase.

Simply put, MCTs are metabolized like a carbohydrate meaning they do not go through the lymphatic system. Instead, these oils go directly to the liver (much like fruits) where ketones are formed and then used for energy in the brain and body.

This process involves much more than is being explained here, however it is good to know what kind of fats you are getting in your diet to allow the most bang for your buck.

Remember, excess calories from any food source can be stored as fat, however WHERE you get your calories from can determine how easily the fat burning or fat storage process occurs.

Think of coconut oils as a fuel that the body knows what to do with and has an easier time converting to an energy source with less wear and tear on the body than carbohydrates, especially processed sugars and fats. You would use the best type of fuel in your car, so why not put the best, most efficient food in your body to allow it to run more efficiently. Again, the easier the source is absorbed (such as with MCTs, especially before a workout to minimize glucose burning and maximize fat burning during our weight/cardio training), the more effectively gains are noticed.

This post isn't necessarily for the person who just adds coconut oil to everything else they eat, but rather for the person looking to see and feel changes. By REPLACING certain fats and carbohydrates with coconut oil you can allow your body to run more efficiently allowing less fat storage and maximum use of excess stored energy aka the energy in fat cells.

Other sources of MCTs include sheep's milk (good luck) and palm kernel oil (not palm oils).

Take Your Time!

Eating takes time, but not near as much time as it takes the body to respond to the food you consume.

Essentially, we all want immediate gratification in life. We want the reward as soon as we complete the task. We want to see someone else punished as soon as they commit the crime. However, just like in the real world, immediate response time is hard to come by. Yes, this does occur in the desire for weight loss.

WHAT!!!??

I know, I know. There is a certain threshold that when your blood sugar dips below that threshold we get the true feeling of "hunger." The longer people go without eating, the lower their blood sugar goes until the body has to begin breaking down proteins to convert to blood sugar; the lower the blood sugar, the more intense the cravings for fatty and sugary foods. The body knows where the necessary calories lie. So then we eat a larger amount of calories then we need to try and "overcompensate" for a lack of energy or low blood sugar. When we consume foods, no matter how sugary and processed, it takes the body TIME to digest food into glucose and respond to those blood sugars, so we overeat.

Highly processed foods spike blood sugar and then insulin is released to respond to the high blood sugar. Easy come, easy go. The blood sugar crashes, so the weight gain is twofold. Not only did we overeat to overcompensate for the low blood sugar levels, but then insulin is released causing a fat storing effect in the body. Insulin quickly crashes the blood sugar level leaving a desire for more – you guessed it – sugary and fatty foods. The cycle can be never ending.

Unless …

Yes, regular meals consisting of minimal complex carbohydrates, proteins, and healthy fats can sustain blood sugar levels and prevent the large crashes and spikes that the average Western Diet usually consists of.

Again, we have all heard this information before and nothing I am saying here is really ground breaking, however whenever I recommend multiple small meals throughout the day to clients, I still get a look like "what for?" This reminds me that we hear so much about food and what we should and shouldn't do that I think we forget the big picture. For example, the Dr. Oz show allows us to expect the body to do work and produce results in a "quick" amount of time.

The latest product I hear recommended is ...

This is again not directly related to insulin or the metabolism, but more so with hunger prevention.

This is where I get frustrated. I understand that a show has to get ratings and ratings are achieved with products and quick answers. Unfortunately to do a show about the body, health, and nutrition and expect anything quick is ridiculous. I feel as though all of the housewives who watch Dr. Oz (or shows like it) and think that by adding ACAI or Goji Berries they will revolutionize their diets and burn fat is annoying, to say the least.

Honestly, as the title of the post states: "take your time." The counselor in me has to recommend being mindful and living in the moment when it comes to eating a healthy diet. Find foods you like and find a way to eat that you don't have to just "make it through to hit your goal," but instead consists of foods and concepts you truly enjoy. This whole "healthy living" thing is a long term process that should be lived and enjoyed. If not, then it doesn't matter what your goal is or why. To think that you can sustain a life you hate for the minimal reward at the end of a long, long road is impractical.

So, for the first time in your life when it comes to results and your body, let's be real. Let's take our time and feed the body like we want to live healthy long term, not just for today, or this weekend, but for life.

#mileycyrus

As a joke in my twitter feed, I have a tendency to put #mileycyrus when it actually has nothing to do with the singer/actress Miley Cyrus. I don't know why I do it, but I think it's funny when things are completely irrelevant and randomly placed together.

I think the TV show *Family Guy* does a good job of this when they do the cut-aways where they mention an idea that is far removed from the topic of discussion, however is funny on its own.

Something else that does a good job of putting two completely non-relatable things together and making a funny combination are the phrases "fat free" and "not a reduced calorie food."

Huh?

How does that work?

I mean, most people assume that by taking a product that naturally contains fat, like ice cream or peanut butter and reducing the fat that the calories would just fall right out of there.

Well, apparently out of our three macronutrients if we reduce one, yet the calories stay the same, then the other two have to increase. More than likely the food industry (who loves the phrase "fat free" or "reduced fat" or more recently "sugar free") will not spend the extra money to add protein to food, so that leaves only one option: sugar!

Here's an example:

Reduced fat Jiff has 190 calories and less fat, but has 16g carbs

Regular Jiff has 190 calories and 7g carbs

Even worse, it may not even be sugar as much as it could be maltodextrin or dextrose (higher glycemic rating than sugar by far). If you look at the reduced fat Jiff one of the main ingredients is corn syrup solids.

#gross!

Yes, what I am saying my friends is that though a chemically altered and packaged product isn't bad enough, they actually have the audacity to remove fat which has its benefits and replace it with more sugar which causes the desire for more "reduced fat" or "fat free" product. Also, if you notice in many cases the "reduced fat" and "fat free" products actually cost MORE.

Ha! Oh food industry, you win again!

Not only do you manipulate people into thinking they are eating a healthier option by removing "nasty" fats, but you replace it with cheaper, more addictive sugar, charge more, and then still have people preferring that overly sweet taste.

It's genius.

I mean very few marketing strategies are as well developed as the hold the food industry has on people's brains. It is as if we have now been raised with these certain tastes and consistencies that are fake and yet are all we know.

I think in one way or another we all know somebody that actually prefers packaged and processed as opposed to the natural and more expensive ingredient food item the by-product is mimicking. In this instance I think of beef. So many people (especially here in Nebraska where we pride ourselves on genetically-altered beef) prefer the taste and consistency of corn-fed beef. When these people are given grass-fed beef, they don't like it.

What!?

I mean that beef only cost me $11.99 a pound and it is chock full of benefits, but you prefer the 80/20 ground chuck fed corn, hormones, and vitamin supplements, fried on the grill with your reduced fat cheese and diet soda?

Sigh... Well, this is where we're at. Just as I have taken the most recent celebrity teen to adult tragedy and thrown it as a tag line on the end of my Tweets, the food industry has joined the two foreign concepts of removing a high calorie nutrient, but yet still claiming that the food is not "reduced calorie."

It really is amazing to me, but yet not near as funny as #mileycyrus.

Got You CORN-ered ...

I eat sugar free, so I consume maltodextrin instead. Wait ...

I eat my veggies every day. Corn on the cob is my favorite ... ah man!

I choose to save a couple of bucks so I use ethanol ... dang it!

OK, I have decided to change my diet so I am eating more fish from the best farm in town ... damn!

Yup, looks like all angles lead to corn when it comes to food, liquid, gas, and overall living these days. I guess maybe I should be thankful that one of the most widely popular items needed by the human species is one that Americans grow very well. I am, however, slightly upset that we have to incorporate corn into absolutely everything these days.

Considering that the molecular structure of corn literally consists of a more concentrated energy source that we are now infusing into everything we eat and drink, it's not such a wonder why people are able to put on weight in excellent amounts.

Really, look it up: corn is like the most concentrated energy source on the planet. I am glad that as a human race we have discovered this energy source. More importantly, I am happier we have GMO-ed it up and processed the hell out of corn to make any product imaginable, all of which in the food world could be the biggest contributor to obesity rather than anything else, ever (sarcasm here).

This is a bold claim some may say, however I ask you to really think about it the next time you are at the grocery store looking at the highest sugar content, most calorie dense products there are. I almost guarantee that these foods contain corn in multiple forms. If the flour doesn't involve cornstarch or the sweetener isn't a CORN syrup, or even corn meal, then at least the carbohydrate derivative maltodextrin or dextrose will be there. Both have very high energy content (meaning calories).

Go ahead, look around. Even if the products somehow do not have some sort of corn product in them, then the fuel it took to ship the food across the sea, across the country, or even the entire world uses a little bit of corn somewhere along the way. I mean God forbid we ride a bike to the farmers market and get fresh food. Not saying that I don't drive everywhere, because I do – I drive a lot – however, I will be the first to say that even I need to make a change for the better.

The CORN industry is HUGE! It compacts more calories into our lives then we as humans were ever meant to have in multiple life times. I could only imagine if my great grandparents who were Germans from Russia were to see the quantities and overall quality of today's processed foods. Even my grandparents were making food from scratch. Then my dad really doesn't cook, so the traditions are slowly dying.

With this idea in mind, just remember that there are some huge companies out there such as Microsoft, Macintosh, Cisco, and BP oil, but none of them can compare to the privatized Cargill which buys almost all of the seed corn produced among other ingredients for almost every processed food worldwide, which means they could literally control the world if they wanted too.

Essentially we are CORN-ered people and I recommend we at least start looking at nutrition labels and know what and how much corn we are getting in our products. I am not here to beat GMO products into the ground, but rather to re-establish how important it is for people to grow or buy local rather than packaged, calorie-dense foods.

Again, just something to think about.

Maybe I'll Start Eating
from the Dog Dish!

Organic food is everywhere.

Let's be honest, if you wanted to, you could spend $10 on a pack of organic, kosher, grass-fed sausages, or 68 cents on a pack of Bar-S hotdogs: your choice.

The same goes with dog food.

I noticed this as I was on the treadmill the other morning watching something on the Food Network. Never watch the Food Network when doing cardio - it messes with you.

Anyhow, so there was a commercial I noticed for Blue Buffalo Dog Food. The claim is that there is no artificial this and fake that, but most notable are the claims on the label that can trump even some of the healthiest "people" food items.

Even at 5 AM on a cardio machine, I had to laugh at the audacity of a company to put more effort into the nutrient content and quality of a pet food over what most food companies are willing to do for human beings.

It's ironic really.

I mean, most dogs have a ten to twelve year life span, so what is an organic, grain-free, non-GMO dog food going to do for the longevity and quality of a twelve year life span? I have three dogs myself and still cannot see the importance of this. Instead, we in America should ask why we don't get this "real" of food. This is in reference to some of the biggest companies in the world too including Subway, with the whole yoga mat bread thing.

Look, for me to get a food item that is certified grain-free, with no added corn or fillers, I have to go to a section of the grocery store where the aisles are paved in gold, or at least should be for the price of some of these things. It is hard for me to understand that to live a healthy life you'd have to pay for, what exactly?

Transportation of food products?

The harvesting of organic material?

Whatever part costs the most, we are willing to pay it to get "novelty" food items, items such as packaged cookies, chips, and crackers that are made with organic material, cane sugar for sweetener, and only use Pink Himalayan salt rather than nasty processed sodium pellets. I know for a box of organic crackers you can pay up to $9 and even then is the air in that box organic, because that's all I was getting in the past.

So, where do we go from here? I mean if there are dog food companies that are willing to harvest, process, and distribute large bags of dog food commercially, how is human food, again packaged, not able to do the same thing without spending more per ounce than any drug dealer would ever get for even the finest product?

These days it is awesome to claim that a product made in a manufacturing plant does not have any corn, wheat, or soy. Even with some of the finest protein supplements on the market they have trouble claiming to be gluten, corn, and soy free. So, how are dog food companies such as Blue Buffalo able to see such a high quality product without sacrificing the integrity of the business and putting a little corn or wheat filler in the mix like most other dog foods?

This radical comparison is to provoke thought and question why it can be so difficult for humans to get this same quality of nutrients. I would like to thank the people who already look for the best food in whole, natural sources such as grass-fed meats, cage free eggs, organic dairy, raw nuts and seeds, vegetables, and berries: food items that are natural and whole on their own. To the people spending large amounts of money on the "novelty" food items that claim to be whole and natural I would like you to question what it is you are actually paying for. The same thing goes for organic dog food. I haven't come across any research to show the benefits, but I guess people feel better when buying it. Either way, the next time you reach for the kale chips, sweet potato puffs, or the cane sugar, organic flour cookies, remind yourself that eating more "natural" usually starts with getting foods that don't have a package in the first place.

In the Moment!

We all need a little inspiration from time to time. Positivity is huge in terms of success. In fact, all we really have is our own thoughts and perceptions, so why not surround ourselves with positivity?

Honestly, think about it the next time you wake up early to get to the gym or attempt to work that second shift for that overtime check. The final product is what we all want. However, it's being in the moment when it needs to matter the most.

I bring this topic up for anybody who aspires to accomplish that goal that is just plain hard. For some people just waking up in the morning is difficult enough. Keep at it and talk to a friend if life just seems overwhelming. As for those who get up, go to work, pay bills on time, and then on top of everything else decide to sign up for a marathon, bodybuilding show, triathlon, work challenge, or anything else extra I say…

"Stay in the moment."

When it comes to accomplishing any difficult goal, sometimes we allow ourselves to be consumed with how much sacrifice we are giving as opposed to the excitement of just living that moment. Take all you runners preparing for the marathon/ half-marathon here in a month. To all of you I ask "how is training going?" If your answer consists of a sigh and a head drop followed by excuses or whining, then again I have to ask: "what keeps you going?" I mean really to those who struggle every… single… day I have to wonder what does it for you?

Is it the fear of failure?

Is it something you actually like however feel that your answer should show stress and fatigue? Really self-reflect here, I'll give you a second.

From time to time I compete in bodybuilding competitions and I know when people ask me how training is going I respond with "OK," because it's something I don't think much about until I am in the moment. When I am "in the moment," not only am I concentrating on the action at hand (muscle contraction, breathing, pushing) but I also think about all those motivational quotes depicting people in Under Armour gear sweating and just getting it done. I put myself in that mindset: the strict, determined-to-finish, and better-than-the-competition mindset. In that moment I know I am doing the best I can. I have to know what I am capable of. When I get back in my vehicle after lifting past exhaustion and way past calorie intake, then I ask myself "was that a good workout?" even though I already know the answer. I was there, I was paying attention, and you could have asked me and I could have told you right then if the thing was going my way or not.

Maybe this post is just for me, or maybe there are others who struggle with being "in the moment." People who get stuck in a mindset of past or future endeavors and negative thinking or comparing their sacrifices to everyone else's end up missing their own life. Many of my clients compare themselves with what they see online, on TV, in movies, books, or social media. Clients see Jennifer Anniston eating a piece of pizza and think that they deserve one too. Little do they know, she hasn't had pizza in six months and her slice of pizza will be just that: a slice. If there are any other issues, then the clients are unaware of what is really experienced. If a client were to see me at a grocery store getting a pizza they might think that all I preach is BS. Again they are not there for the many days without processed sugars or flours.

Go out and get whatever you want to get, eat what you want, and do what you want, just stay in the moment and find pleasure in it. If it is a degree in school, find interest in your studies. If you want to complete a weight loss challenge, find joy in the challenge and what you are learning about nutrition and yourself. If you are deciding to raise a child and are stuck in the moments of difficulty such as staying up all night or changing diapers or the lack of social life, well, this one should be a given, but enjoy your child. Duh.

I don't know about my readers, but I needed this. The motivational quotes can only go so far until they just aren't enough to push you through those tough times. Maybe with a real point of view about my own struggles and challenges you may get just the right piece of motivation needed to get up in the morning, at least enough to alleviate that isolated feeling that sacrifices needed to achieve personal goals can bring.

Fats and Carbs: Not the Modern Day Bert and Ernie!

MMM … fats!

They are my favorite. I mean, don't get me wrong: carbohydrates can be fun, like pure sugar or a good sweet potato, but nothing has the satiety of a handful of almonds, scoop of peanut butter, avocado with cheese, coconut oil, or olive oil. Honestly, carbs without fats are just boring. People eat candy which is nothing but high fructose corn syrup and dextrose usually; however, there's no long-term satisfaction. It's just sugar… yawn.

NOW, a big doughnut, that's what I'm talking about. Deep-fat fried batter with chocolate frosting that is that diabolical combination of sugars and fats. Just like any other processed and highly coveted food item there is usually a combination of carbohydrates and fats. The carbohydrates give that immediate pleasure in the brain and the fats give texture and density aka "mouthfeel" as the food industry puts it.

Birthday cake without fats is nothing more than a pile of flour; however the cake without flour is a pile of fat. The two need each other to be the pleasurable combination that tastes so good, but ends up being so bad!

For anybody wanting to cut some stubborn body fat I recommend giving fats and carbs a divorce. Yes, the combination of bread and butter or pasta with cheese, cheese and crackers, oatmeal with cream, high carbohydrate cereal with 2% milk, or any other traditional combination sounds enticing and innocent, however makes simple digestion difficult.

"On the other hand, the foods to avoid if you are trying to lose weight include: fried foods, chocolate fudge, alcohol, potato chips, all desserts, corn syrup, buttered popcorn, ice cream, pies and breads/pastas."- Michael Kennith Author of <u>Just Add Good Stuff</u>

1. The body digests carbohydrates first, then fats.
2. Carbohydrates turn to blood sugar starting in the mouth, then into the small intestine, into the blood stream, pulled out by insulin, and then used as muscle glycogen, brain functioning, and stored in the liver.
3. This energy will be used up before the body uses any fat stores, so keep that in mind you high carbohydrate eaters.

As my readers know by now I am not necessarily a strong fan of the "calories in versus calories out" belief. In fact, certain people who are insulin sensitive suffer with this mentality and store more body fat through carbohydrate-rich meals than a person who is just genetically leaner for whatever reason. With this in mind, think about eating that sandwich which has bread (carbohydrates) and meats and cheese (fats). The carbs digest fast and cause an insulin release, while the fats in the meats and cheeses will store as excess calories and end up maintaining body fat or possibly even putting some on.

When carbohydrates are digested, a byproduct, glycerol phosphate, is produced which then attaches to the free flowing fatty acids already in the blood stream. This then forms triglycerides which are the large fat deposits that sit inside adipose tissue. So, fats by themselves are great energy sources, however, in the presence of carbohydrates, triglycerides are formed and then, well, it's just not good.

One thing that happens is that triglycerides have been shown to prevent leptin (the hunger suppressing hormone) from crossing the blood-brain barrier to do its work.

Again, leptin is the gatekeeper of fat metabolism, monitoring how much energy an organism takes in. It surveys and maintains the energy balance in the body and it regulates hunger. If leptin is absent, feeding is uncontrolled and relentless. So, with this in mind, keeping leptin levels high allows the body to regulate as it was meant to, rather than be overridden by simple carbohydrates driving hunger.

This is best achieved by keeping the consumption of the two macronutrients separate.

Example:

Regular meal: toast with peanut butter and 3 whole eggs.

What I see: highly processed Carbohydrates with fat, good protein source, but again, more fats.

What could allow for easier digestion? Oatmeal with egg whites or protein powder.

Why? Complex carbohydrate with a solid protein source, either slow or quick digesting depending on the next activity time.

So, give your body, blood sugar, hormones, and overall lipogenic activity a rest and separate your fats and carbohydrates just like when your mom used to ask you to separate your clothes.

You never really wanted to do it, but it made finding the clothes you needed early Monday morning much easier.

Separating carbohydrates and fats can take the stress off of the metabolism and help people choose healthier foods. This is because most high carbohydrate foods are packaged with processed fats and are overly stimulating.

You've Lost That Hungry Feeling!

"I'm hungry."

It's a phrase we hear often. I'm not sure if people are actually hungry, or if the availability of food and the pleasure food can bring these days is to blame for the increased use of this phrase.

Some people just say it as a way to say something, I think.

Watch the next time a quiet moment occurs while studying with friends and someone says, "I'm hungry." In many cases, I think we're bored. My mom used to question me all of the time about this. She would ask if I was really hungry or if I was just bored.

This confused me.

I mean, for a child to turn to food items because you're bored? I remember thinking about this question as a child and being perplexed.

Bored, huh?

Well, then I never knew how it actually felt to be hungry. It's like that urge to eat was always bad and "hunger" was something that got in the way of living a life I wanted to live.

Growing into my very awkward adolescent years, I felt that "hunger" all of the time. I mean true hunger and yes I do mean all of the time due to the way I figured out how to lose weight. I would restrict calories and completely negate the physiological response of my body needing calories as nothing more than a slight headache or inconvenience. Don't get me wrong, my physical symptoms such as dizziness, fatigue, trouble concentrating, and difficulty sleeping and working out, even moving at times became very problematic, but I always stayed motivated. I was in control of my food and I could do anything.

I think it was in season seven of <u>The Office</u> where Will Farrell comes onto the scene as the new boss after Michael Scott leaves the show. Well, he struggles with eating and states that he conquered obesity. One episode depicts him sitting next to a vending machine and with a voice in the background stating that "once you conquer obesity you can do anything."

144

That is exactly how I felt in high school when I would go two to three days without eating a single thing. It was a high unlike any other. It was like this nauseous yet euphoric feeling drove me day to day to see how far I could push it. I would stand up sometimes and brace myself against the wall because I was seeing black spots. There were more than a few times when I would end up on the ground (thank God never in front of anybody), and I would wake and be confused and disoriented. I would always brush off the incident as minor.

Needless to say, I lost weight – a lot of weight. I think in 6th grade I weighed 215 pounds and by my junior year in high school I was down to 170 pounds. So, during those critical growth and development years I was starving myself in an attempt to gain the life I saw everybody else having. So, again, I was HUNGRY. This feeling occurred so much that I just thought this was how I was going to live my life.

Through various situations in my life I have attempted many different styles of eating and have found that eating consistent, non-processed and nutrient rich foods in moderation is the way to go.

Surprise!

So, then what does all of this have to do with this post title?

This question is critical to any weight loss plan, or improving on body image, cravings, and mental health. Hunger is a response the brain interprets from the hormone levels of insulin (among other factors) to let the conscious part of our brain know it is time to decide on what to eat.

For me as a child, I was never truly hungry and I ate food for pleasure, because I didn't NEED it like a hungry person does. Now, when truly hungry, such as when I became an adolescent, I enjoyed egg whites, broccoli, almonds, spinach, salmon, and oatmeal, all foods that when I was a child were dull and grossed me out. This is how I know I am actually hungry these days.

Ask yourself this simple question: am I really hungry?

If not, and any time you desire a snack consisting of high sugar, high fat, or some fried and processed food by-product, then

145

again you are not truly hungry. Don't even mention starving. If you are truly hungry you need nutrients (carbohydrates, fats, protein with vitamins and minerals) in their most easily digestible and absorbable forms. Fortunately this can be found in whole food sources. Do not be fooled: if you are studying late into the night, pulling a second shift, feeling stressed, or anything out of the ordinary, then yes that desire for sweet and salty snacks is going to be more enticing than when we get regular sleep, regular foods, and have lower amounts of stress. So, be prepared for this. Tell yourself: "I am not hungry. I am just looking for something to help stimulate my overworked brain." Sugar releases dopamine and the food scientists know where to gear advertising and how to make some of the worst foods seemingly innocent.

Remember to find pleasure in other areas of your life rather than drugs, I mean *food*. (Sorry, Freudian slip.)

Eating "Healthy" Doesn't Equal Weight Loss ...

OK, so I have decided to turn my life around, eat organic, and lose some of this stubborn body fat.

I am going to Whole Foods and spending $150 a week on the richest, freshest, most natural foods I can get my hands on. Well, I mean some of the items are packaged, but don't worry, they are made with organic cane sugar, coconut sugar, agave nectar, date sugar, maple syrup, or honey, so I should be good.

(TWO MONTHS LATER)

What the heck! I have been eating as rich and organic as possible and still no weight loss. I mean, before I was spending $70 a week at Wal-Mart, but now I literally am spending a fortune and still no difference.

Well, this is frustrating. I even follow all of the "healthy" recipes on Pinterest. I use bananas instead of ice cream: the recipe where you take four bananas with honey and cocoa powder and blend it up, and still no weight loss, increased energy, or all those benefits I hear so much about. I guess I might have to start going to the gym, or just go on an all protein no anything DIET.

The above scenario is one that I hear from people all the time. In fact, I myself have fallen victim to many of the fallacies of "organic" and "all-natural" food sources. Truth be told, and I have mentioned this many times before, even if sugar is organic, minimally processed, from natural sugar, or God forbid, honey, you are still consuming a carbohydrate source, a quick energy source that in turn will cause a spike in insulin and therefore trigger a fat storage response.

It is that simple. I do not care if you replace every food item in your grocery cart with organic and raw, if it contains sugars of any kind (yes this includes fruit), then losing that stubborn body fat will not be an easy task. I promise.

You will hear about people who lose weight by switching to organic or minimally processed foods, but in many cases it is because they might have started working out, or they started eating more fibrous foods and therefore eating fewer calories, or some other correlation. Simply replacing all of your calories with the exact same number of "organic" calories is no way for weight loss to occur.

This concept is one that frustrates people. Many of my clients figure that by spending large amounts of money on food automatically means it digests more efficiently in the body, or magically can pull calories out of the body. This has never worked and never will.

I personally get frustrated with this concept because I could care less how "green" your smoothie is if it contains thirty grams of fructose. Even worse is adding honey to food products which should already be sweet enough. I mean I would rather see an artificial sweetener added if you NEED sweetness. An example is a bowl of oatmeal, which is great. It's slow digesting and has tons of benefits. However, when any recipe calls for honey or bananas to be added, then I have to interject and say to add a few packets of an erythritol/stevia mixture for sweetness without adding calories.

Simple.

I am not even going to get into the conversation of natural this and benefits of that because people want to feel good of course; however, they want to look good as well.

Much of the time people argue that there are all of these benefits in fruit, however any nutrient you find in a fructose concentrated product you can find in a vegetable, usually in larger amounts for less total sugar.

For you fans of Food Babe on Facebook, I have to call her out because many of her recipes are misleading and assume that something is "healthy" because it "comes from nature." It just isn't that simple. When people think it is, they feel that they can eat as much as frequently as they want. Yes, if you are going to consume a coconut milk ice cream replacement instead of a bowl of actual ice cream you can be slightly "healthier," but that is not what occurs.

Instead people find something, run with the basic "this is healthier than that" view point, and eat it all of the time.

Food Babe describes various "healthy snack" ideas that all involve some sort of sugar (organic and raw of course) or large amounts of fat (again unrefined). It's a good start, but people are getting confused on what and how much they can still eat of these "treat" options.

So be wary of all of those healthy options at your local "health" food store. Honestly, I was checking a few weeks ago and besides some organic cinnamon or pasteurized almonds, I really didn't find anything too extravagant. I mean cereal is still cereal and candy is still candy no matter how expensive it is.

Finally, a Way to Suppress My Immune System! - Said No One Ever!

This isn't 100 percent true. Actually, there are many people with autoimmune diseases where the body begins attacking itself who need a suppressed immune system. There are also people who receive organ transplants that need suppression of immunity so the body will not reject the organ.

Suppression of immunity in organs needs to occur in special circumstance that most of us should never have to face.

As for everybody else, the immune system is what keeps us alive and well. Without it we would all have to be like the old Jake Gyllenhaal movie Bubble Boy. (I bet people forgot he was in that.)

So, take a look at this:

2-acetyl-4-tetrahydroxybutylimidazole aka THI, which is responsible for the caramel coloring in sodas.

(Apparently they can just put caramel coloring and not name the actual chemical name.)

Not only does this "caramel coloring" cause your soda to remain brown, but research has also shown a correlation with suppression of the immune system. That is about all it's good for in the soda world: an immunity suppressor simply used to color our beverages.

Well, that scares me.

Maybe because years ago I drank diet soda like a fiend and I still wonder about the long-term damage I did to my body. I mean, by lowering my immune system, I put myself at risk for getting a disease and being unable to fight off that disease in a timely manner.

This was my drug of choice … dang!

Now, combine the idea that the caramel coloring in combination with the average amount of regular soda consumed by Americans, or three hundred seventy-nine twelve ounce cans per year, not only reduces immunity but has a number of negative effects on the body. One major consequence of sugar is that it prevents the full break down of nutrients in the body. This can lead to a "leaky gut syndrome" or IBS or gastric problems, whatever you want to call it.

Now we have a two headed dragon where the body's defenses are down and the sugar in the soda is affecting the breakdown and absorption of everything from vitamins to minerals to proteins.

These are just a few of the negative effects of the ol' soda pop. There are numerous other reasons why a person shouldn't consume these containers of sugar, carbonation, and phosphorus laden water. Any ailment related to immunity or needed nutrients for recovery and growth of cells is now directly affected by this world-renowned product. Sugar increases acidity in the body as well.

Many people read the beginning of this and decide to drink Gatorade or fruit juice instead.

Wrong!

Don't waste your time on these "alternative" sugar drinks because the "sugar" in them is still just that: "sugar." Yes, the chemical composition can be considered a bit different such as glucose being processed and broken down early on and fructose, or the sugar found in whole fruits, being broken down in the liver. However, both are very readily available energy sources that honestly have no benefits to the average non-athlete.

I have to remind my clients about this all of the time. Sugar in any form (honey, maple syrup, cane syrup, or fructose) is still just that: a sweet and easily broken down and digested carbohydrate source. Even foods made with agave nectar, which is considered "more nutritious" due to its low glycemic rating on the glycemic index, are just other forms of sugar. However, once again we have been deceived by marketing. Agave nectar is nothing more than 90% fructose and therefore has to process through the liver but is still too concentrated to be of any value.

To conclude my original point, stay away from soda the best you can, by that I mean don't touch it EVER. When cooking or looking for a sweet alternative, you can save a lot of calories by enjoying some sugar-free beverages from time to time.

Lowering your Cholesterol Starts with a Sweet Tooth-dectomy!

Cholesterol is a funny thing really. Funny not in the sense like I am, which is hilarious, but more so in terms of how beneficial it is for our body and yet has such a bad reputation.

First off, there are the HDL (or high-density lipoproteins) and then there are the LDL (the low-density lipoproteins). Generally speaking, HDLs are good and LDLs are bad. HDLs take triglycerides out of the blood which is why they are good. LDLs have a tendency to build up in the arterial walls restricting that good blood flow.

OK, now with all of that established I want to remind people that cholesterol occurs naturally in our bodies and is essential for everything from hormone levels to regulatory homeostatic functioning of body processes. Remember, homeostasis is the neutral state we want our bodies in.

So, if we consume foods that are high in processed sugars and low in fats like everyone was attempting to do in the 90's, then we are theoretically putting ourselves at risk for heart disease.

Also, adding "sweeteners" to products adds that little bit of stimulation people are seeking.

When we remove the fats from foods or consume a diet rich in processed carbohydrates and low in fats and cholesterol our body's natural ability to make this cholesterol, which it does, has to work that much harder to compensate for the sugary foods consumed. The body does this to keep a balance in the body, or a ratio of cholesterol that is needed to sustain homeostasis.

So, in layman's terms, high carbohydrate foods with either fats taken out, or processed sugars and flours added, actually can be a cause of high cholesterol more so than eating naturally-occurring fat could ever do. Obviously, I am still opposed to man-made fats, such as hydrogenated oils, but the naturally saturated fats and both mono- and polyunsaturated fats are there for a reason.

WE NEED THEM!

Heart disease is the number one killer.

Even my own father told me at my wedding reception last year that the doctor stated his cholesterol was high and recommended medication right off the bat!

Wrong!

God forbid we make some changes to our diet!

In talking to my dad and knowing his very standard and traditional ways, I know that many of his meals consist of nothing but carbohydrates. Not in large quantities like I would do, but nonetheless he would consume Cheetos while at work or bowls of cereal for a quick dinner. These meals that are high in refined carbohydrates, combined with his age of 62 are huge factors for putting someone at risk for heart disease.

What I told my dad to do was to incorporate more lean protein sources, not to be scared of nuts and legumes, and if he wants a steak or some red meat with a higher saturated fat content from time to time to go ahead and have it. Those bowls of cereal have to go, as well as the refined carbohydrates. Essentially what I recommended to my father was higher in fat and cholesterol; however his numbers improved over the year.

Weird, huh?

No, not really. There is tons of research on this topic. Unfortunately, many doctors still like to get paid and they don't get paid off of people controlling their own blood sugar levels by reducing processed carbohydrates in their diets. No, doctors get paid off of the pharmaceutical companies. So, instead of changing your diet, a statin drug can be prescribed to do the trick.

Something to remember whenever taking a cholesterol lowering drug is that the side effects can be severe because when cholesterol levels are artificially manipulated the brain, which is 60% cholesterol, takes a big hit in its ability to think and process. There are reports of higher instances of suicide for people on cholesterol-lowering medications.

So, without getting too preachy here, go ahead and lower the amount of processed sugar, white flour, or any refined carbohydrates in your diet and get back to foods the way they were meant to be eaten: whole, minimally processed, fat rich, and protein dense.

Enjoy that butter with your meal or that coconut oil on vegetables. I say go ahead with that steak on Friday night, but hold off on the dinner rolls or dessert. For an alternative dessert for your sweet tooth, I recommend using heavy whipping cream and a little Truvia artificial sweetener to make yourself a high fat, very low carbohydrate dessert if you are craving something indulgent. The effects of small changes over time will show on your latest blood work. When the Dr. asks what you did to change your diet, you can say you were eating "the good stuff."

Cheers to the Weekend!

Normally, when it comes to nutrition and health I figure you should stay away from alcohol at all costs. Honestly though, besides the extra calories there is a lot more to making beer than just a fancy bottle!

Yes, there is also a nutritional connection here!

First off, yeast: who would have thought? Yeast is very interesting due to the fact that its purpose is to break down sugars using alcoholic fermentation. The one-celled organisms are anaerobic (do not use oxygen) and break sugar down into CO_2 and ethyl alcohol (ethanol).

So, yeast makes the alcohol.

Yeast essentially does the same thing when it comes to making bread, which I always assumed was its more common use.

In bread-making, yeast has three major roles: to leaven the bread, strengthen and develop gluten in the dough, and to contribute to flavor.

Maybe the jobs of this single celled fungus, in which alcohol is produced as a by-product, are the same no matter if we are making bread or alcohol. It appears since both need yeast to work appropriately that the sugars are converted to an alcohol-like state, which is a more efficient way to inject carbohydrates into your system. Nothing like getting those carbohydrates broken down and absorbed quickly, except for the sudden insulin release and ultimate weight gain… dang.

Think about what yeast would do in a body that consumes hundreds of pounds of sugar a year. What fermentation processes are occurring inside of our bodies?

Is my body just a hub for free-radicals?

Am I just begging for cancer by consuming food and drink laced with yeast that is fermenting inside of my body?

Or is there another way to look at yeast?

Candida is a form of yeast, and a very small amount of it lives in your mouth and intestines. Its job is to aid with digestion and nutrient absorption but, when overproduced, candida breaks down the wall of the intestine and penetrates the bloodstream, releasing toxic by-products into your body and causing "leaky gut syndrome." This can lead to many different health problems, ranging from digestive issues to depression.

If you remember, in earlier posts I discussed the blood-brain barrier and how foods containing gluten can penetrate this barrier and cause mental health problems by allowing toxins into the brain. When the body becomes imbalanced or you consume too many enriched, enhanced foods that cause over growth of bacteria, this can also lead to some pretty bad symptoms. Also, there is a direct connection with our brains and our stomachs. So if the GI tract isn't working properly, then we aren't.

Doctor recommendations in treating certain GI issues are to provide the body with what it needs (or in this case what it doesn't need) by reducing the consumption of the more complex carbohydrates such as grains, beans, fruit, pasta, and potatoes to only one cup a day. Eventually this type of diet change causes overgrown bacteria to die out.

Seriously folks: unfortunately the reaction between yeast and sugar is not a pretty one and the internal workings of our body really take a huge hit when we begin to ferment foods in our digestive tract! This reaction can even affect skin appearance.

Yes, there are medications and stuff, but among the other 45,000,000,000 reasons to reduce or eliminate sugar I think that just cutting it out will never hurt you. I would bet money that reducing sugar and processed, refined grains could result in you feeling better both mentally and physically. Leave the yeast to the brewers and allow me to walk you through the idea that when something is wrong with the gut or somewhere in the billions of reactions occurring in the GI tract that a change of diet should be step number one.

You see it every day!

We are so dependent on processed, refined foods rich in ingredients like yeast that we continue to overconsume them despite negative results. The idea of giving up sugar and refined carbohydrates scares people more than any Zombie Apocalypse ever could (had to think of something scary).

Lazy!!

Just one more rep!

Just one more set!

How about just one less cookie, or a whole lot less, well, everything.

Have you ever read a nutrition article that recommends some kind of sweet tasting fruit or diet drink, bar, or powder that is supposed to be satisfying and lead to weight loss benefits?

I know you have.

I think back to Dr. Oz a few years ago when ACAI juice was all the rage. People were paying $4.00 for these chubby little concentrated juices simply because they were associated with fat loss. Unfortunately for those who were looking to lose weight and spent a fortune on juice, when you squeeze the fruit and only get the juice out, you have now lost most of the benefits and you are left with nothing more than a beverage with more sugar per ounce than SODA!

So, yeah, go ahead and put the juice back on the shelf.

It does not matter if the juice is 100% or not. Just stay away. Again, we hear what we want to hear and a good-tasting juice is easier than eating a plate of broccoli with salmon and adding exercise. Remember that sugar in fruit processes through the liver, storing more efficiently than any other carbohydrate source. This pushes fatty acids out into the blood stream to make room in the liver for the processing of these fructose sugars. If you have been paying attention, then you realize that this elevates your triglyceride levels. All due to concentrated amounts of, yes, fruit, specifically juice.

Dang!

Also, you never actually lose fat. Instead, your fat cells shrink. So get rid of the "burning fat" concept right now. While we're on the subject, the idea that our bodies even want to shrink our fat cells or lower our subcutaneous fat is false and there are many internal processes in play to help override any "diets" or exercise programs.

Once again we hear "burn fat" and boom, we are sold, despite the fact that these claims are erroneous!

I know as a society we think there is some external product or routine that can just undo the damage we have done to ourselves over years of bad choices. It is because we are lazy and hear what we want to hear, which is usually the easiest, tastiest route. This route is also the least effective if not downright detrimental. This isn't our fault as humans, though. I mean our brains do not like stress. Instead, we rely on things to alleviate that stress like easy diet methods or some product that can do it for us.

> "Whew, I feel better knowing there is something
> that can help. Now back to my pancakes and bacon.
> I'll pick the product up on the way home."
> - Defense mechanism of the conscious mind

This is where I come in. I do the research, utilize my health background to interpret information and combine it with my counseling skills to help people apply what is true to their own life. Understanding basic concepts about food and nutrition does nothing more than provide a base. The tricky part is putting the knowledge into practice.

Again, there is no magic pill, bar, drink, diet, routine, secret fruit, magical massage or purple dragon that can save you from yourself. Trust me: I work with people who struggle with addiction all day, almost every day. Your own self-destructive tendencies will take you out quicker than anything else ever could.

Yes, though food addiction is not YET classified as a treatable disease I can tell you assuredly that it is most definitely an epidemic. No, make that pandemic. With this being a fact, and yet the diet and weight loss supplement business being in the billions annually, there is something I am missing here. I mean, if weight loss pills work (and they must because we the media doesn't lie to us), then why are so many people becoming so overweight, sick, and depressed? Why is there an increase in occurrences of metabolic syndrome, obesity, and diabetes?

I mean, the pill can erase anything, right?

Screw the stats, this takes a behavior change!

The funny thing here is that when you begin to look into how bad things like sugar, trans-fats, even refined and processed grains are, the results are always the same.

It is all bad.

In fact, look at some of the most successful "diets". They usually involve kicking sugar and lowering or eliminating any refined grains. In many instances, fruit is also considered poison. Also, when it comes to anything packaged, look that stuff up. I mean, the manufacturers are selling a product, not food. If they were selling food, then it wouldn't be able to sit on the shelf for months, sometimes years, before being pulled. But hey, we all have to make a profit, right? Well, yes, but the food industry, which is pretty much comprised of ten major companies and over six hundred thousand packaged food items, is one of the few businesses that make more money as the years go by. They continue to develop ways to cheapen and de-nature food more, and more, and more, until what is left is so refined and filled with additives that it is now a thing, not a food.

According to the book, <u>Fat Chance</u>, oranges are not sold as a commodity on the stock market because they get old and moldy within days. However, orange juice with all of its preservatives and processing (yes even the 100% stuff) is sold on the stock market. Interesting how the food isn't worth very much, but man we turn it into a refined product and bam we have gold!

But who cares?

Honestly, day to day when it comes down to it, who really cares? The stats are there and the articles are out. Nobody thinks McDonald's is the fountain of youth, just like your morning doughnut has literally been deemed one of the worst foods ever invented. French fries are thrown on your plate as a side as if the extra thousand calories of starch and boiled oil is nothing. Sodas get bigger, people buy value meals worth thousands of processed and denatured calories because "it's a deal." I mean, who cares about what the stats say if you do not internalize the importance of the information presented.

Nutrition is nothing more than "eat this, not that" and here's why ... blah blah blah.

Dietitians and nutritionists have all of the knowledge yet many of them are overweight themselves, so then why would I listen to you when you can't do what you recommend. You tell me to consume more green leafy vegetables and lay off the breads and sweets, yet you have a candy dish in your office!

It is a waste of time to go see the doctor with a nutritional deficiency, not because they aren't smart, but because they treat symptoms. That is all. The medical model is to treat the symptoms based on what is taught. You can't just write a prescription for a B vitamin because somebody is depressed - that makes no money. However, they do have some Prozac and Lexapro that will fix you right up.

Again, I work with a few doctors for some severe ailments that need further medical examination, but overall when it comes to a nutrition solution you need a nutritional counselor!

What!?

Yes, a counselor that has a strong background and certification in nutrition that can help you with knowledge as well as the behavior modification needed to make a lifestyle change and put these nutritional ideas into play. Supplements and nutrition do not change your behavior or what it is you internalize and hold on to day to day. No, you NEED behavior modification, otherwise expected prognosis of your relapse from weight loss isn't sustainable.

Look, all I'm saying here is that we've (yes we all have) gotten nutrition and diet and exercise wrong thus far, but someone is profiting from it and it's not the people paying the money or taking the supplements or even buying the most organic of organic foods. We the people are getting convinced through lies and manipulation that the way to make a change is to pay big bucks and sacrifice everything we love to get our weight down to a level where we get compliments.

A counselor helps you rebuild the most powerful machine in the world, the brain! Your thought process about food can be rewired and reconfigured (aka behavior modification) with time, sessions, practice, knowledge, and application. Yes there is a sacrifice, but the way you were living before was a sacrifice. You were sacrificing your true inner peace and happiness for what? Pizza, a doughnut, your sugary coffee drink? All of these items are drugs: they don't help, and you don't need them.

Again, the research is there and there is a lot of it, but people want a pill to change everything. It all starts in the brain that has been developing since we were inside our momma's belly. Counseling sessions not only involve reflection and knowledge but a better understanding of your own thoughts as well as coping skills that assist in the challenge of turning down that (enter favorite food here). The change starts with the first session and you can never look at food items, diets, exercise, and supplements the same way. You will get nutritionally mature.

Try something different, something that can benefit you for the rest of your life without spending your life paying for it.

SYNDROME X!!!!!!!

There is a new movie coming out this summer about a syndrome that is killing people, literally leaching their very souls with a sweet and simple aroma. It sounds f-ing scary! Worse than the first time I saw <u>The Ring</u> in high school with my then girlfriend Jenna for whom I had to act tough. I am going to make a confession: I was scared and could not sleep that night!

Whew, I feel better.

Jenna if you read this, do not judge the confused, awkward, and pimply-faced kid I was. It wasn't really my fault. I mean, I wasn't always the nicest person and usually tried to act tough.

If anything, I was high on sugars – or even worse –- due to my restricted calorie diet in high school, maybe my blood sugar was low, causing me to have trouble thinking, be anxiety ridden, have trouble sleeping, and be moody, among various other things.

No, this isn't about me and my ex-girlfriends watching scary movies. I think Rach would appreciate that, or she would just laugh at me. Either way, I better move on.

SYNDROME X aka Metabolic Syndrome is no joke, people, and unfortunately it is called this because there is no other way to describe so many different symptoms in one disease.

I'm talking personality disorders: antisocial personality disorder and border line personality disorder, all of which lead to struggles in everyday life that medication cannot touch. I'm talking about trouble thinking or concentrating, moodiness, lack of motivation, poor job performance, yelling at your spouse and immediately regretting it. These are just a sample of the mental health ailments caused by Syndrome X. Some physical effects of Syndrome X include diabetes, hypertension, heart disease, and stroke, basically all of the things that will simply kill you if left untreated.

This monster is a nasty one and it can creep up on anyone. The worst part is that it moves into your life like a ghost and begins to influence your decision making ability, your motivation, your mindset, even your activity with friends. Everything is affected by the precursor effects of Syndrome X.

One day you decide to have a doughnut instead of oatmeal and fast food instead of your salad. The next day you do the same because those foods tasted good. A couple of weeks go by with high stress, long hours, and minimal sleep and you find yourself eating prepackaged meals or drive through for almost all of your caloric intake. Let's not forget the sugary coffee drink at Starbucks or the snack at the mini-mart on top of everything else. Also, due to your busy schedule you just can't make it to the gym and find yourself sick, overweight, and just feeling blah.

I will admit the foods taste good and getting that little bit of extra time to yourself by skipping the gym can seem beneficial at first. However, time continues to pass and you go to your next checkup and your stats are all off. Your blood pressure is up, blood sugars are elevated, and triglycerides are up.

"Doc, what is going on?"

"I am having trouble sleeping, my sex drive is low, my clothes don't fit, I have no motivation, and I don't do anything anymore. I think I need an antidepressant."

(Freeze frame with frightened look on the patient's face.)

No sir, you have just been stricken with Syndrome X!!!

(Dun Dun DUUUUUUUUNNNNNN)

"But why me?"

Honestly, sir, you feel this way because you have been eating like crap, not exercising, and living an extremely high stress lifestyle. Essentially you are killing yourself slowly and it is with the "comfort" foods you turn to.

So yes, this disease can creep up on you and it gives you all of the warm, good feelings of apple pie, cakes, cookies, pizza, and ice cream, but after some time and constant consumption of these products without restraint, BAM! The body simply cannot keep up the fight.

So what do we do to prevent this pandemic from consuming the world? Well, we eat one ingredient, whole, plant-based foods, lean protein sources, and fat that comes from plants or fish and is not whipped up in some tub or manufacturing plant.

Yes, these foods may not provide the type of comfort you are looking for in terms of immediate reward, but they will provide you with long-term satisfaction and, oh what's that word? Health!

Look, Syndrome X aka Metabolic Syndrome is a syndrome or collection of various health ailments brought on by the introduction of the "Western Diet" rich in sugars, processed fats, refined grains that are void of nutrients, high fructose corn syrup, dextrose, maltodextrin, and fructose added to products that forces the body to go into survival mode. In this mode, the body has to push fats out into the blood stream because we keep feeding ourselves foods so rich in processed carbohydrates that our one liver we have is being over-worked. Again, I have said this a thousand times, but let's at least make an attempt at resolving an issue that we created in a lab and now is spreading throughout the population. The worst part is that it is controlled by the choices we make every day.

Efficiency of Foods ... Guaranteed Way to Lose and Keep Off Weight!

Here's a diet for you: it's called the Efficiency Diet. Essentially you eat the most efficient foods you can find. For example:

Breakfast: 1/2 Cup steel-cut oats, 5 oz. salmon, and 1 cup spinach leaves (raw)

Meal 2: 1/2 Cup quinoa, 6 egg whites

Meal 3: 1 Cup black beans, broccoli, and 5 oz. salmon

Meal 4: 1/2 Cup steel-cut oats, 6 egg whites, spinach leaves

Meal 5: 1 Cup Steel-cut oats, 6 egg whites, kale

Meal 6: 5 Whole eggs, spinach leaves

Meal 7: 1/4 Cup walnuts (raw), 1 tbsp. Chia Seeds, 4 whole eggs

By the way, this is my diet!

This would be an example of eating efficient foods. Other foods to add would be different types of wild fish, grass-fed beef, different varieties of plants, berries of varying colors, oatmeal, steel cut oats, raw almonds, pumpkin seeds (pepitas), and other seeds (quinoa, sunflower). Pretty much if it grew from the ground, swam wild in rivers or oceans, was plucked from trees, or was naturally raised and fed on a farm, it is nutritionally efficient.

What is efficiency? Well, here it means getting the most bang for your buck, the most nutrients for your calories. I could waste 100 calories on prepackaged processed crackers, or I could get more than one cup of black berries for my 100 calories. With the berries I also get antioxidants, fiber, vitamins, and minerals, all in an easy to absorb form. With the prepackaged, processed 100-calorie crackers I get white flour, processed oils, and who the heck knows what else.

So, why have people not heard about this diet?

Simply because it is not a "diet" in the traditional sense. It is a way to live healthier, more EFFICIENTLY and longer while enjoying activity and vitality. This is essentially a gift from God and should be accepted as such. These foods are raised from the ground to build and nourish the body. They are not meant for food scientists to grow in mass quantities, genetically modify, sugar coat (among other things) and then sell for a profit. Nope, not these!

The processed and modified way of eating has been tried, and, hopefully, is on the downhill slide. (I am an optimist.) The rate of heart disease, cancer, and number of deaths associated with processed food items is killing more people than any natural food could ever undo and make healthy again. In terms of straight calories, according to the package, processed and genetically modified foods can be seen as something useful. However when it comes to bioflavonoids, micronutrients, and macronutrients (all in balance), we are essentially moving away from the farm and losing the efficiency of foods right along with it.

If anyone has seen the show The Walking Dead, then they can make this connection: "don't leave the farm, people!" As long as everything was going ok in our world living off the farm why did we have to go and try to make things better? Why could we not just stay put and avoid disease and imitation food-like products. We have diseases and illnesses that this world has never seen before popping up all of the time. Malnutrition was supposed to have been solved with GMO but because of our reliance on food-like substances instead of actual food it is still alive and well, unlike its consumers.

So, what do we do with our current "Western diet"? We essentially toss it out, start over, and try getting something fresh every single day. Then we can move to multiple times a day until we are eating raw and unprocessed food items. Education about nutrition and the detrimental effects of processed foods is available and is becoming more accessible.

I just want to remind people that this is not going to be easy; however, it is going to be useful and will be a lifetime investment in something of which you only get one: your body!

26 Days 'til Christmas ...

Actually, I started the countdown to Christmas as soon as Halloween was over.

In fact, I wanted to put up Christmas decorations the day after Halloween to enjoy as much of the seasonal activities and atmosphere as I could before we take it all down in January.

This being the weekend of Thanksgiving where families get together, enjoy good home cooking, and maybe a little shopping to buy gifts for the ones they love (do not get hurt going to Wal-Mart for a $93 TV), I wanted to say what I am thankful for.

Here we go ...

I am thankful for family, friends, food, and blessings.

I am also thankful for the body's ability to process neurotransmitters from the food I consume so that I can think positively and clearly when needed.

Some people might think that is an odd thing to think about and be thankful for when there are so many other, more obvious, things in the world to appreciate.

I say: not true.

Even when people are constantly putting large quantities of food by-products in their bodies, the body is still able to efficiently break down, distribute, and absorb the nutrients needed to properly function. This is especially important in the brain which controls everything.

People need to be more appreciative of their bodies and what they constantly go through, even though we still expect them to run as efficiently and effectively as possible. No other machine in the world could take the damage day in and day out and continue to run as efficiently as our bodies do, let alone at all. Think about drug addicts, severely obese individuals, the elderly whose work conditions exposed them to deadly chemicals throughout their lives, cancer victims, and people who drink day in and day out for years with no elevated liver enzymes.

Let's say, for example, that you decided to consume turkey, mashed potatoes and gravy, sweet potato casserole, dinner rolls, pumpkin pie, ice cream, whipped cream, stuffing, butter, cheese, green bean casserole, and various other traditional Thanksgiving items in large quantities and then awoke the next day expecting to feel the same as you would any other day. There is the potential that you woke up feeling lethargic, more sore than usual, and maybe a little more anxious or depressed. Did the drive to save some money wake you up early for Black Friday shopping? Did you need a sugary coffee drink to get you going, or what I like to call a "sugar-coma remedy?"

Why on earth would people think that they could stuff themselves with food for the entire day before and then awake feeling both physically and mentally fit the same as any other day? When we give the body something stimulating, or an excessive amount of processed, sugary foods (yes flour, mashed potatoes, corn, and actual sugar all would count here), it experiences a rebound effect that may not come across nearly one fraction as appealing as the taste of the food did going in.

I'm talking about the physical symptoms such as multiple bathroom breaks, dry mouth, loss of sleep, discomfort, agitation, lack of motivation, sadness, roller coaster moods, boredom, and lack of stimulation from simple pleasures including being around the ones you love. All possible symptoms are due to our own conscious decisions to overeat and the body's subsequent need to process and digest such food items.

My suggestion is keep everything in moderation and allow minimal amounts of processed and sugary foods. I know that during the holiday season this is not always an easy task due to the availability of and encouragement to eat said processed foods. View your body as your best friend. Do you want to take advantage of your best friend and consume crappy foods that will hurt it, or do you want to turn down processed foods so you can continue to feel good, confident, and motivated?

Remove your emotional attachment to food (especially holiday food) and view your relationship with food the same this time of year as you would any other time. The food may be differently colored, it may remind you of nostalgic days gone by, and may be more available to you now, but your mindset still controls what and how much goes into your body. By doing this, the body will more ably process the nutrients it needs from whole food sources instead of experiencing negative symptoms as a direct effect of consuming processed foods.

Personally, I cannot consume sugar and still expect to remain "lean," even on a semi-annual basis. I understand that my reaction to these foods is poor; however, as foods continue to become more processed, many more people will be insulin sensitive just like me. I lose my mental clarity and motivation when I indulge. My own mental health and overall quality of life is as serious and real as any diagnosed physical ailments.

Bodybuilding!!!

If you are looking for a worthwhile activity that helps you focus your time and attention on your physical self, may I suggest joining the bodybuilding circuit?

Just follow these simple steps:

1. Consume a lot of calories and lift really heavy weights forcing your body to respond with muscle growth.
2. About 2-3 months out from a show, start to consume fewer carbohydrates, more vegetables, less fats and begin doing a daily cardiovascular activity.
3. The day before the show, drink water, shave, spray tan, and get a haircut.
4. Next thing you know, you're on stage posing in front of a whole bunch of people you do not know in a tiny little garment of clothing.
5. Pick up your trophy and go home to start the process all over again.

Sounds easy, right?

Wrong.

I am in no way an expert on the ins and outs of bodybuilding, however I have had experience with a few shows and have worked with and around people who have participated in both amateur and professional shows.

To see these contestants up close, it would seem that everyone on stage is the pinnacle of health. They look amazing. I bet they eat vegetables, lean protein, and just enough fats for mental health. I bet they workout 2-3 hours a day, every single day of their lives. I also bet these people never get tempted by sugary treats and abstain from such indulgences, which is why they look so good.

Again, wrong.

I don't want people to glorify the guys and girls they see in the weight room working out for a show as something any average person could not obtain through diet, exercise, and healthy habits. I want every day Joes and Josephines to know that the people you see on stage sometimes struggle more with food and having a healthy relationship with food than the average person.

Take my wife for example. She eats when she is hungry and for the most part she could care less about a "cheat" meal. One day she could eat a Hot Pocket, the next day a spinach salad with chicken breast and walnuts. She bases her decisions on what is available and her body telling her when it is time to eat. My wife does not glorify food as do I and therefore her relationship with food is a healthy one. She does not covet, designate a cheat meal, or even associate the holidays with processed and sugary foods of her youth. She simply eats when hungry in moderate amounts and then stops when no longer hungry.

My wife does not currently participate in any fitness competitions; however she works out and knows the benefits of living a healthy lifestyle. I would match my wife's common sense approach against any person on stage where the emotional attachment to food is concerned.

My point here is that if you have a goal of competing in a bodybuilding, fitness, or bikini show, give yourself enough time to make changes before signing up. Assess yourself and your relationship with food to make sure you are able to pass the test and recover properly afterward. Seek advice from a nutritionist or nutritional counselor to understand the mindset needed to ultimately obtain the lean structure you see in magazines and posters, and then do what it takes to accomplish your goals.

Less than 5% of the general population will ever compete in a bodybuilding/fitness show. Considering an overweight kid from western Nebraska with genetics from "big" parents can sculpt his body with nothing more than diet and exercise, anybody can do it. My recommendation is to not approach your goal of doing a show as unobtainable. Instead approach it like any other goal you set for yourself. Consult with a coach and surround yourself with other like-minded people looking to compete. Again, assess yourself and your quality of life to remind you what is most important. Truth be told, there is no special talent or skill involved in competing in shows, just hard work, discipline, sacrifice, and dedication.

If you want it, go out and get it. Maybe I will see you on stage this coming summer. Look online for local bodybuilding/fitness shows and decide what it would take to formulate a plan and achieve that goal.

Merry Christmas Ya Filthy Animal!

"Christmas time is here" (as sung by the Peanuts gang)!!!!

So, what's next?

I have already hung the stockings (I did that, like, November 15th), put up the tree, put up lights, bought my Christmas candy (to look at), planned my trip home for Christmas, and even started watching horrible Christmas movies on Netflix. (<u>Christmas in Handcuffs</u> for example, plus we already watched all of the classics.)

So, what else could I do to pass this holiday cheer around for all to enjoy?

SING!

No. I better not, considering I have been told I might have the worst singing voice ever.

Holiday party time is right around the corner, which could keep my cup full of holiday cheer … that and Sirius XM radio's holiday channel playing nonstop in my car since early November.

Yes! I love holiday parties. There is always food, decorations, and people having a good time and trying to pack an entire year of "joy" into one night of drinking and horrible Christmas sweaters.

If you understand the blog posts by now then you know I have an issue to talk about and nothing can be left to "simple" pleasures.

Let us do a little math.

Your basic metabolic rate is equivalent to 3,000 calories. It takes 3,000 calories to keep your body at a steady weight while maintaining enough energy to perform all of the body's necessary functions.

So let us say you eat 3,000 calories a day to maintain your body weight. Then you go to a party where tables are loaded with drinks and cookies and breads and your favorite nachos (the kind with green and red chips). Now, say, at this particular holiday party you consume 4,500 calories. The next day you work out extra hard and end up burning 3,500 calories, an extra 500 over your ideal metabolic make-up. That is awesome, BUT you still have an extra 1,000 calories from the night before in the form of processed and fat storing goodies. Let us say you go back to your regular schedule of eating exactly what you burn, but then along comes another party, and another, and then Christmas Day is really bad, then New Year's Eve, then New Year's Day, then ...

Now you are into January and you are a few pounds overweight without even trying. My problem here is not with the parties, per se, but with the excess amount of "life" that is at the parties. I'm talking booze and food. The food is always sugary, breaded, fried, cheese-covered and processed, and the booze is always, well, available.

So, what is my holiday survival guide for eating healthy?

Eat right, eat small, blah blah blah. You know this already, but still you choose not to do it.

This is where I recommend taking a good hard look at your decision-making process and why you continue to justify eating such processed and nutrient-devoid products, such as cookies and nachos. You are at a party with friends and coworkers and yet you need more stimulation from excess food and drink? No. That is nostalgia, or the emotional part of your brain reacting and that is certainly a weak point for many (including me).

We remember the foods we grew up eating such as fudge covered Oreo's, sugar cookies in the shape of Santa, traditional breads, mom's homemade something, even the green and red nachos which taste no different than the nachos that are available year round.

Instead, have a bottle of water and do your best to minimize excess and enjoy yourself without food at the many holiday celebrations you are invited to. (I always assume my readers are the popular ones.) I know that I was able to make it through many celebrations this past year following my own rationale to feel good. I learned a great deal about how much I rely on food and drink to make an event entertaining for me. I was able to remove the need for extra stimulus and have a good time for what it was: a social gathering.

So, for this January, reward yourself and stay the same. Add muscle, or lose some body fat. Get a hold on that need for the external stimulus of processed goodies available in excess this time of year.

I also recommend looking up healthy recipes online to know that what you bring to the party is safe. That way you won't look as though you are missing out on all the "fun" everybody else gets to experience.

But if you do find a way to make those green and red nachos in a healthier version, let me know because they always look so GOOD!

Soy? Really?

When I was going to school I wanted to be a dietitian so badly. I thought their job would be so cool. I mean, you are the expert in telling people what to eat. You have the last and most authoritative word when it comes to nutrition. I remember sitting in my nutrition classes looking at the RD's with admiration and envy.

Imagine naïve Luke just sitting in his chair looking at the sky daydreaming, "I wish oh I wish upon my shiniest star that I could be one of them."

Then I grew up!

Look, I'm not here to say I am the final expert on anything related to nutrition and health, but I am old enough to realize that nobody really is. Truth be told, everybody is so completely different. With the millions of chemical interactions that occur in the body when food or drugs are consumed it is just baffling how we could even be similar at all. Some people are sensitive to this and others to that, but either way there are general rules one must follow when recommending food to others.

This is my beef. (Ha ha beef instead of soy, get it?)

Much like when I was a naïve young college student and I looked up to the RD's in my program, I now realize the world puts too much confidence into what these people have to say. Honestly, way too much!

For clarity on my point go to your grocery store and ask for the dietitian and have a somewhat modern day conversation with them about macro nutrients. Don't even get into supplementation or effects of foods on blood sugar, interactions with specific fats, and packaged versus raw or organic foods. I think that you may be surprised by the reasoning behind why some foods are chosen. I'm telling you, there is just too much faith put into what these people have to say.

For another little piece of clarity on how a dietitian isn't really that useful, turn your radio on to a country station and listen to the endorsement from a dietitian about SOY of all things.

SOY?

I personally thought that at this point in our culture we had moved on from our ignorant faith that soy is useful for anything other than filler. The "protein" in soy isn't even a "complete" protein. Just like every other plant, it lacks amino acids and therefore cannot replace all of your meat sources unless you know what to combine it with. I mean, I guess I will start my argument there. The protein content in soy is bunk.

Secondly, do you know you can't digest raw soy? Yes, soy has to be processed to be able to be digested by the body. In fact, the process starts by using hexane or other solvents to remove the oil (which can be sold as cooking oil or oil to be added to other processed foods), and then we take what's left over (defatted soy flour) and either combine it with other proteins to make animal feed or wash it with water to create soy protein concentrate. I must also note here that soybean oil is used in processing foods and is rich in Omega-6 fatty acids. One hypothesis is that this overabundance of fatty acids is responsible for brain disorders and increased amounts of Omega-3 fatty acids are needed for brain health (Psychopharmacology, Joseph Wegmann, 2012).

Soy protein concentrate becomes the source for two forms of soy that are even more processed: TVP (or textured soy protein that can be produced through a process called extrusion) and SPI (soy protein isolate, which can be produced by making the soy protein concentrate more solubilized). SPI is used in many low-fat soy milks.

You have to look at those labels!

1. Soybean crops are heavily sprayed with chemical herbicides, such as glyphosate, which a French team of researchers have found to be carcinogenic.
2. Soybeans naturally contain "antinutrients." Traditional fermentation does destroy these antinutrients. However, most consumers of soy do not consume fermented soy, but consume unfermented soy, mostly in the form of soy milk, tofu, TVP, and soy infant formula.

3. Soy's antinutrients are so interfering to the body's homeostatic functioning that drinking just two glasses of soy milk daily provides enough of these compounds to alter a woman's menstrual cycle.

4. In fact, infants fed soy formula take in an estimated five birth control pills' worth of estrogen every day.

Oh soy, why!!!????

So, I guess what I am asking here is why, as a dietitian who is supposed to be like the government authority on nutrition, would you endorse this product?

Well, besides the money I guess.

I understand that soybeans equal huge money because the food companies found an easy-to-grow crop and then decided to put it in all foods. The food industry is literally powerful enough to change how and what we eat. We have all had the SOY pulled over our eyes and we didn't even see it coming!

Well, here we are, getting recommendations from "experts" to eat more soy when the negatives just can't outweigh the minimal amount of benefits. These are benefits that we could find and eat in other nutritious vegetables, all of which are preferred over gross soy!

So, I guess I should thank God that I did not become a dietitian and give in to what the government aka "the food industry" wants me to believe. Instead, I like to look at the facts and go back to the way things were, without soy that is.

I mean, after all, the people who make money on the product have to put warnings on the product stating it contains soy.

Think about it!

Weight a Minute!

According to physics, weight could simply mean mass which is a property of a physical body which determines the body's resistance to being accelerated by a force and the strength of its mutual gravitational attraction with other bodies. (Yawn ... sorry physics just isn't my thing).

According to science and engineering, the weight of an object is usually taken to be the force on the object due to gravity.

According to most women it's a bad thing.

According to drug dealers weight equals money.

According to the nutritionally inclined community, weight is nothing more than a number and a gauge as to what class you might be in a competition or will help determine what size gym clothes you need to buy. Overall it isn't viewed as good or bad.

Honestly, I would like to take a stab at weight here and remind people that what we weigh is the force with which we are being pulled to the Earth by gravity. When we step on a scale, the scale is able to measure this number, but in space or anywhere that lacks gravitational pull, your weight will drop. Does that make you feel better?

Many people will weigh themselves until the batteries run out on their scales. I know this because I was guilty of this in high school. I starved myself to hit a certain number no matter how sick I looked doing it. This makes no sense now, but that's what I did. Honestly, what does that mean: if I step on the scale, weigh myself, and don't like the number, but like how I look? Then am I supposed to continue to desire change?

I mean, when I weighed 285 pounds I could tell people that I weighed 285 pounds and they would say "oh that's big," but then when they see me weighing 265 with less body fat, people think I have actually gotten bigger because I am more defined. This is how muscles work.

So, why do we focus on weight again?

Oh yea, because that is somehow the universal standard of whether a weight-loss diet or workout regimen is successful or not. The way I see it, the proof is in the pudding, and by pudding I mean the product that comes out of a difficult situation or sacrifice.

I am going to take this a little bit deeper than I need to here, but Viktor Frankl himself said that despair equals suffering minus meaning. So we need to find the meaning in a tough situation to allow for the suffering to be worth it, otherwise it turns to despair.

Think about it.

OK, so what is the meaning of weight again? Who cares?

What is the meaning of hard work and sacrifice? Ahh, there is the question.

In most cases I would like to say that hard work and sacrifice is fun, but it isn't. Instead you need to find an appreciation and day to day satisfaction in what you do to best stay on track with whatever your goals are in life.

As for me I am going to dust my scale off because it is hiding in my closet beneath some old shoes. Maybe I can sell it on Ebay or something.

Perceive Happiness

The middle of December can mean anything from happy thoughts of holiday gatherings to times of loneliness and sadness. It can also spark thoughts of relaxing and displacement of worry about ... possible calorie intake?

Your perception of the world is what you make of it and though you cannot always control your environment, your perception of that world is what you allow to affect you.

For example, someone may say that the weather has been cold and nasty outside and complain and grumble about the icy roads, slick sidewalks, and the thick layer of frost on our cars every morning.

Or

This person could view snow and cold as the appropriate change of the seasons that brings about moisture and cleanses the air of all of the pollen and bacteria that form outside without the extremely cold temperatures.

In fact, in the book <u>World War Z</u> written by Max Brooks, the winter time is the safest time of year due to the zombies freezing or becoming immobile due to the extremely low temperatures. (They would eventually thaw out again in the spring and summer months.)

What about processed food, Luke? Does that have a place?

Ah, now there is a question.

Honestly, yes.

Do we need it?

Maybe.

So then what are the positive side effects of processed food-like items such as high fructose corn syrup, gluten, and hydrogenated oils?

To be honest, the population on this Earth would not be sustainable without the invention of the aforementioned food by-products.

Are these food-like items considered healthy?

Again, not really, but they have allowed food to be developed, processed, and preserved for long periods of time in bulk to feed the world what it needs: macro nutrients. Yes, the vitamins and minerals have their necessary benefits, but without the calories from GMO (genetically modified) foods, a large amount of the population living right now would have to die off.

What I am saying is that everything has its place in life. The good needs the bad to be good and the crappy times in life need to have the good ones to make life worth living.

I look to the book <u>Man's Search for Meaning</u> written by Viktor Frankl where he describes his days in a World War II Jewish concentration camp. This man didn't know if he was going to live or die or if the loved ones he was separated from were alive. He worked entire days not knowing if he was going to get fed, watered, or just die working like so many of his companions around him did daily.

This puts life in perspective and peers deeper into the superficial that the Western Society glorifies with over consumption and greed.

Just look at what we glorify for Christmas: presents galore, high calorie food items, booze, candy, Christmas lights, wrapping paper, etc.

All of these are highly consumable items that have the potential to interfere with the important factors in life such as, oh I don't know, family and friends!

Just as I recommend eating moderately you can expand this idea of moderation and live your life and save the excess for a time that you deem necessary.

Maybe the holidays are your necessary indulgence, which is fine. However, make sure that you are prepared for the overindulgence with budgeting, planning, and a designated time for exercise. Again, this is much like consuming a healthy diet. It's weird how those two correlate.

During this holiday season view the snow as beautiful and appreciate just being able to spend time with friends and family. Forget about all of the expectations or societal pressures to over purchase and over consume to satisfy the need to have more.

Expectations for the Holidays!

With Christmas right around the corner, I expect these next couple of days to be full of happiness, excitement, and relaxation with friends and family.

With this expectation in mind I am assuming that the entire time spent over the next few days will be full of fun and excitement. However, we all know that that is not necessarily true, especially when going back home and sitting around for hours with family members. This is in no way a bad thing, however it is not necessarily stimulating especially if you are used to busy work days where there is hardly time for a break.

When we visit relatives, there is a feeling of comfort and nostalgia that causes people to expect so much more when really we end up getting bored in some way and looking for stimulation. That stimulation or boost we are looking for to keep the seasons merry and bright is found in the form of food and drink, excessive food and drink at that.

Christmas is the one time of year where even the healthiest person will make an exception to his diet. The commercialization and overabundance of food lying around may also increase that feeling of needing stimulation. Also, look at the fact that nostalgia, or foods and drinks eaten traditionally throughout life, touches on an emotional level of comfort and consumption. Those foods may remind people of that feeling.

Well, if one cookie reminds you of Christmases past, then maybe ten will really get your happy memories a flowing?

Next thing you know you find yourself on the couch at 5 PM dozing off because the sugar rush and excitement of opening and giving gifts has passed and the conversation wasn't enough to keep you interested. (Also Monopoly in my house usually gets started up and we all know how long and tiresome that can be.)

Maybe I am wrong.

Maybe I can only speak for myself.

I know that clients of mine consider the holidays stressful partially due to the traditional overabundance of processed and sugary foods. The mindset to overconsume is harder to ignore on this one special day, or week for some.

My recommendation for this next week or weeks before Christmas is to live in the moment of the holidays. Keep expectations about the future to a minimum and enjoy conversation with friends and family for what it's worth: a good conversation. Remind yourself that yes the baked goods and excessive amount of food tastes good, however do I need the third piece of pie, or does that Oreo ball NEED to be eaten, even if it is the last one on the plate?

Maybe by this time next year, with a consistent change of mindset about foods, you will be healthier and more comfortable with food and it will no longer CONTROL you. Rather, let food be a side character in an old episode of your life that is no longer a bother.

Christmas with the Meiers!

Each and every Christmas it's the same!

Wake up… eat!

Open presents… eat!

Engage in discussions… while eating of course!

Then finally we have the Christmas dinner, so eating commences.

When do we stop?

For my family, stopping to enjoy the little things doesn't happen and ever since I can remember Christmas celebrations have been about excess.

I'm not saying that all of the holiday food is a bad thing. I honestly thank God and feel blessed that my family is able to have so much and that we have the excess to spare. However, there is also a point where celebration turns into overindulgence which leads to discontent and eventually into feeling miserable.

It all starts with waking up and eating my mom's traditional Christmas casserole made with eggs, cheese, bacon, and a bread crust. (She only makes this for Christmas.) Then we follow that up with cinnamon rolls and then cookies all come out to be displayed.

Eating healthy is great and challenging yourself throughout the year to eat healthy is important. Now, the real challenge is to stay clean throughout the holiday season or any time period of elevated emotions, nostalgia, or traditions. This is something I have never done before; never even considered actually.

I figured it was impossible to go an entire Christmas not having any cookies, sweets, candies, breads, or drinks.

Well, I am proud to say I did it this year!

Yes! I went an entire trip home (Christmas Eve, Christmas day, and even the day after with all of the leftover food) without any of the baked goodies my mom and aunt are so good at making. In fact, as of writing this blog post I have gone twenty-one days eating clean once again.

But wait…

Why sacrifice one of the best days of the year just to complete another self-imposed challenge?

Sacrifice? Who said anything about sacrifice?

Honestly, I feel as though I was actually able to enjoy the holiday. I was fortunate enough to be able to spend time at home with my wife, brothers, aunt, cousins, mom, and dad.

I engaged in conversation and shifted my focus to appreciate the small things of the holiday season. I looked at all of the delicious-looking foods on the table and decided that they would remove the focus from where it needed to be in this rare time of togetherness.

Would I have enjoyed eating the cookies, fudge, candies, cinnamon rolls, breads, pies, ice cream, and various other sweets at the time?

Of course, silly! However, very quickly after consuming the sweets I would need more, and more, and more to satisfy the unending desire I have for sugar and processed, nostalgic foods. Plus, with the idea that everyone overindulges during the holidays I feel as though it would have been justified.

Again, I know myself and my own personal relationship with food. I decided to remove this external stimuli and enjoy the people, conversations, and internal gratification that we were all able to be together, instead of eating too much by 3 PM and laying on the couch miserable looking for that next high, or in this case, cookie.

Trust me, if I can make it through the holidays, a time where I of all people justify eating poorly, without eating a single goodie, then anybody can. Remember, I have sugar in my genes. I was the overweight twelve year old who would eat entire large pizzas, trays of cookies, and impress friends and relatives with the amount of food I could still put away.

Even earlier this year I was glorifying food and minimizing the negative impact that processed food had on my physical and mental health. At the time I needed that drug and thought there was no way I could live without it.

As for Christmas 2013, it is in the books and my wife and I made it back to Lincoln safely, and then it was back to life as we know it.

I encourage you to find balance with your nutritional choices and to remove the focus of weight-loss.

Epilogue

The writings you have just experienced are what my perception of nutrition is thus far. I find it very interesting that there are people who write books about a specific theory based on the knowledge at hand and are still preaching the same idea years later with new, more relevant information available. Again, I've never considered myself the expert on anything. I'm just a curious person who studies, reads, researches, and counsels others through their mental health problems. I believe the world can incorporate a healthier tone to life with a broader approach to nutrition instead of watching Dr. Oz and learning about some plant and its specific root extract to help ward off cancer. Instead, I figure that the antioxidants and phytonutrients found in vegetables are also going to keep me healthy and able to ward off diseases just fine.

As a people, we make things too complicated. I feel as though we want to make things difficult, that way few people can understand things and it leaves the ones who made it difficult to understand them in a position of power. This gives power to people who appear smart when really they are nothing more than con men. Maybe this is a stab at politics, or maybe I believe that the food industry and government are sitting too close together and that change will never be allowed to occur no matter what happens.

No matter what happens as long as profit margins stay high. As long as people continue to buy the food available and packaged and do not make a choice to grow or develop their own food, shop the local farmers market, or buy from the outer walls of the grocery store rather than the "forever shelves."

So, as my concept of nutrition and health dovetails with counseling, behavior modification, and mental health, then I believe we need to concern ourselves less with the government and more with our individual choices. If the food industry and government want to handle the difficulties of an industry full of processed and sugary goods rather than invest in health, nutrients, and longevity of a quality life, then that is their prerogative.

We are the people, and we are in charge. We are the decision makers and we are the ones who can influence what is available at the store rather than be at the mercy of "what tastes good." "What tastes good" has been genetically modified to taste as such. To think otherwise is ignorant. I want people to read this collection of writings and do as the title of the book says and think.

Consider that the body is nothing more than a set of chemical reactions that happen to digest, absorb and distribute the nutrients where they need to be and then excrete the waste out. Once all of this occurs, then whatever it is you decided to eat that day can either cause problems such as inflammation, headaches, aches, pains, and trouble with thinking clearly, or leave you satisfied, healthy, relaxed, and minimize stress and inflammation.

The choice is and always will be yours. You can choose to consume the sweet candy instead of the bland vegetable. You can choose to do the right thing in life or to take the way that benefits you the most. The choice is what we have as a people and though the right choice isn't always as clear, just ask yourself: who is this benefitting? Just who does it benefit if I buy a box of Pop Tarts? The sugar and white flour combined with copious amounts of other processed and rancid ingredients doesn't help me one bit. I guess the $4 I spent on this over-advertised and over-refined product benefits none other than the company that made it. Thank you Kellogg's, or I guess I should say, you are welcome for taking my money, giving me an insulin spike or short high, and leaving me feeling empty and alone. All of the good drugs leave people feeling like crap: it is in their nature.

So, with this collection of writings from the perspective of a counselor, my goal is to not only educate people about nutritional facts like a dietician or nutritionist, but to challenge readers to take a look into why we do these things to ourselves when the detriment is clear and affects our well-being. I want to challenge my readers and followers of my blog posts to do better, not forever, just for today. As long as you can say I tried my best today, which can include slip-ups, then you did yourself a favor. Again, get the black and white, all-or-nothing thought process out of your head right now. There is simply no room in your mind when there is...

Something to Think About ...